College Vegetarian Cookbook

Quick Plant-Based Recipes Every College Student Will Love

Delicious and Healthy Meals for Busy People on a Budget

Tiffany Shelton

Copyright © 2020 by Tiffany Shelton.

All rights reserved.

No part of this book may be reproduced in any form or by any electronic or mechanical means, except in the case of a brief quotation embodied in articles or reviews, without written permission from its publisher.

Disclaimer

The recipes and information in this book are provided for educational purposes only. Please always consult a licensed professional before making changes to your lifestyle or diet. The author and publisher shall have neither liability nor responsibility to anyone with respect to any loss or damage caused or alleged to be caused directly or indirectly by the information contained in this book. All trademarks and brands within this book are for clarifying purposes only and are owned by the owners themselves, not affiliated with this document.

Images from shutterstock.com

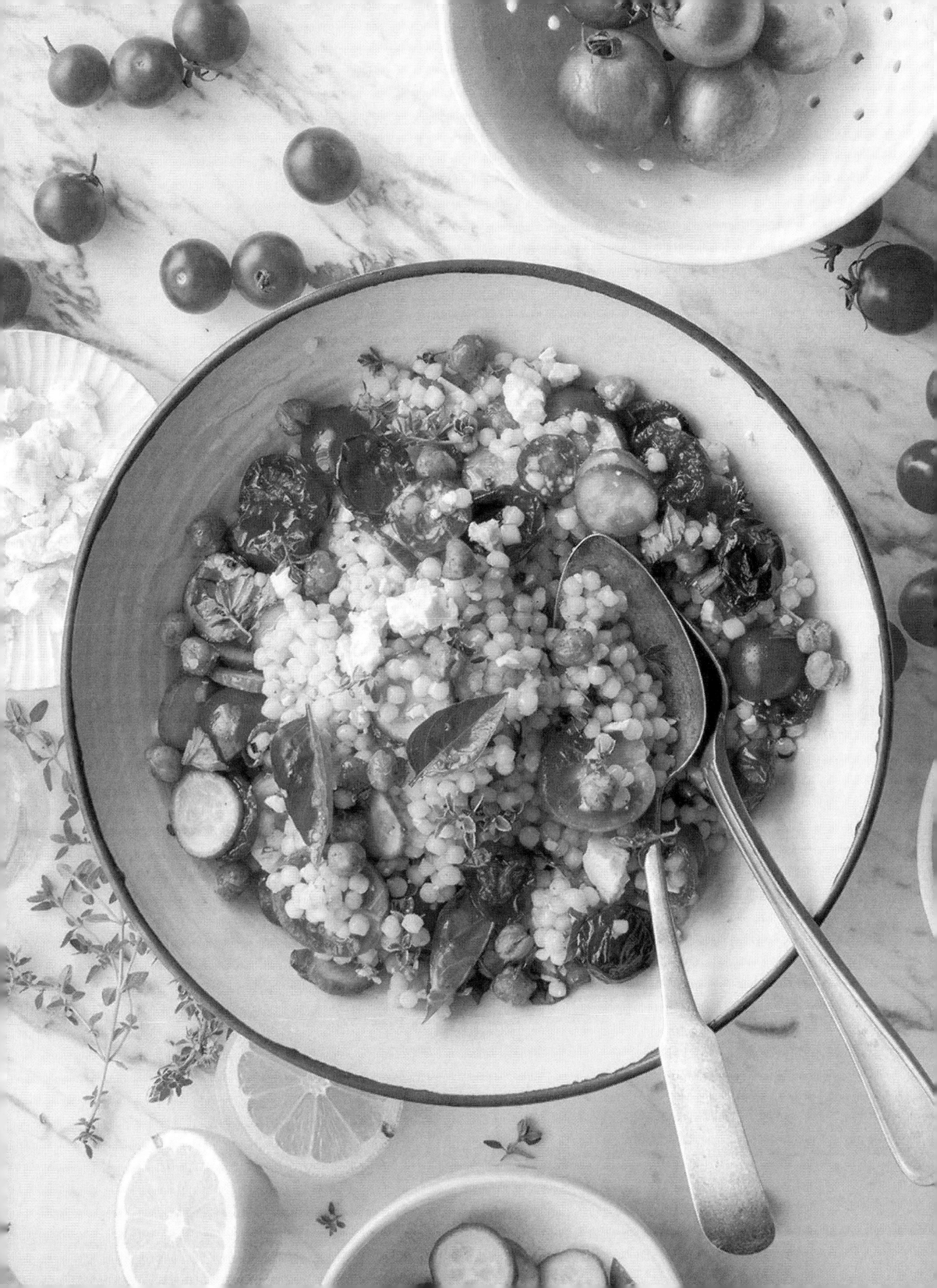

CONTENTS

INTRODUCTION 6
CHAPTER 1. Vegetarian Basics for College Students 7
- Key Ingredients and Nutrients of Vegetarian Kitchen 7
- Avoiding Nutritional Deficiencies 8
- Methods of Cooking Vegetarian Food 9
- Useful Tools and Equipment 10
- Making Your Vegetarian-Student Pantry 11

CHAPTER 2. Three-Week Simple Vegetarian Meal Plan 12
- Week 1 12
- Week 2 13
- Week 3 14

CHAPTER 3. Easy and Healthy Vegetarian Recipes for College Students 15
BREAKFAST 15
- Baked Eggs with Herbs 15
- Green Chickpea Flour Pancakes 16
- Student Tomato Omelet 17
- Breakfast Egg Muffins 18
- Egg-Free French Toast 19
- Coffee Breakfast Pudding 20
- Oatmeal with Almonds and Cherry 21
- High Calorie Oatmeal with Cinnamon 22

LUNCH 23
- Avocado Toasts with Hummus 23
- Tri-Colored Lunch Bowl 24
- Buddha Mix 25
- Spicy Veggie Wrap 26
- Lentil Bowl with Tomatoes and Garlic 27
- Bell Pepper Salsa 28
- Pearl Couscous with Lemon 29
- Corn Pasta with Brown Butter 30

SNACKS & QUICK BITES 31
- Simple Garlic Bread Snack 31
- Potato Chips 32
- Crispy Cheese Sticks 33
- Bell Peppers and Hummus 34
- Perfect Movie Popcorn 35
- Low-Calorie Kale Chips 36
- Crunchy Roasted Edamame 37
- Toasted Pumpkin Seeds 38
- Almond Oat No-Bake Energy Balls 39

SANDWICHES, SALADS & DRESSINGS 40
- California Sandwich with Grilled Veggies 40
- Grilled Cheese Sandwich 41
- Sandwich with Egg Salad 42
- Greek Cheese Sandwich 43

Wild Rice Salad with Pomegranate, Pistachio and Persimmon 44
Bulgar Wheat Salad with Chickpea and Pepper 45
Broad Bean Salad with Barley and Mint 46
Lentil Salad with Avocado and Feta 47
Warm Salad with Cauliflower 48
Soft Tahini Dressing 49
Lemon Mint Dressing 50

SOUPS & STEWS 51
Chunky Chickpea Soup 51
Moroccan Carrot Soup with Cilantro 52
Cold Cucumber Soup with Dill 53
Fresh Tomato Avocado Soup with Basil 54
Hearty Potato Stew 55
Indian Stew with Peanuts 56

MAIN COURSES 57
Cream Cheese Leek Risotto 57
Broccoli Pesto Fusilli 58
Noodles with Carrot and Sesame 59
Linguine with Mushrooms 60
Marinated Tofu with Peanuts 61

DESSERT & FRUIT-FOCUSED MEALS 62
Sushi with Peanut Butter and Jelly 62
Apple Dutch Pancake 63
Delicate Banana Pancakes 64
Baked Banana with Almond Butter 65
Strawberry Cheesecake Toasts 66
Raspberry Vanilla Cream 67
Coconut Muffins 68
Splendid Cherry Ice-Cream 69
Awesome Chocolate Mousse 70

DRINKS & SMOOTHIES 71
Bracing Coffee Smoothie 71
Vitamin Green Smoothie 72
Strawberry Grapefruit Smoothie 73
Inspirational Orange Smoothie 74
Simple Avocado Smoothie 75
High Protein Blueberry Banana Smoothie 76
Ginger Smoothie with Citrus and Mint 77
Strawberry Beet Smoothie 78
Peanut Butter Shake 79
Chocolate Oatmeal Smoothie with Peanut Butter 80
Hearty Peach Shake 81

CONCLUSION 82

Recipe Index 83

Conversion Tables 85

Other Books by Tiffany Shelton 86

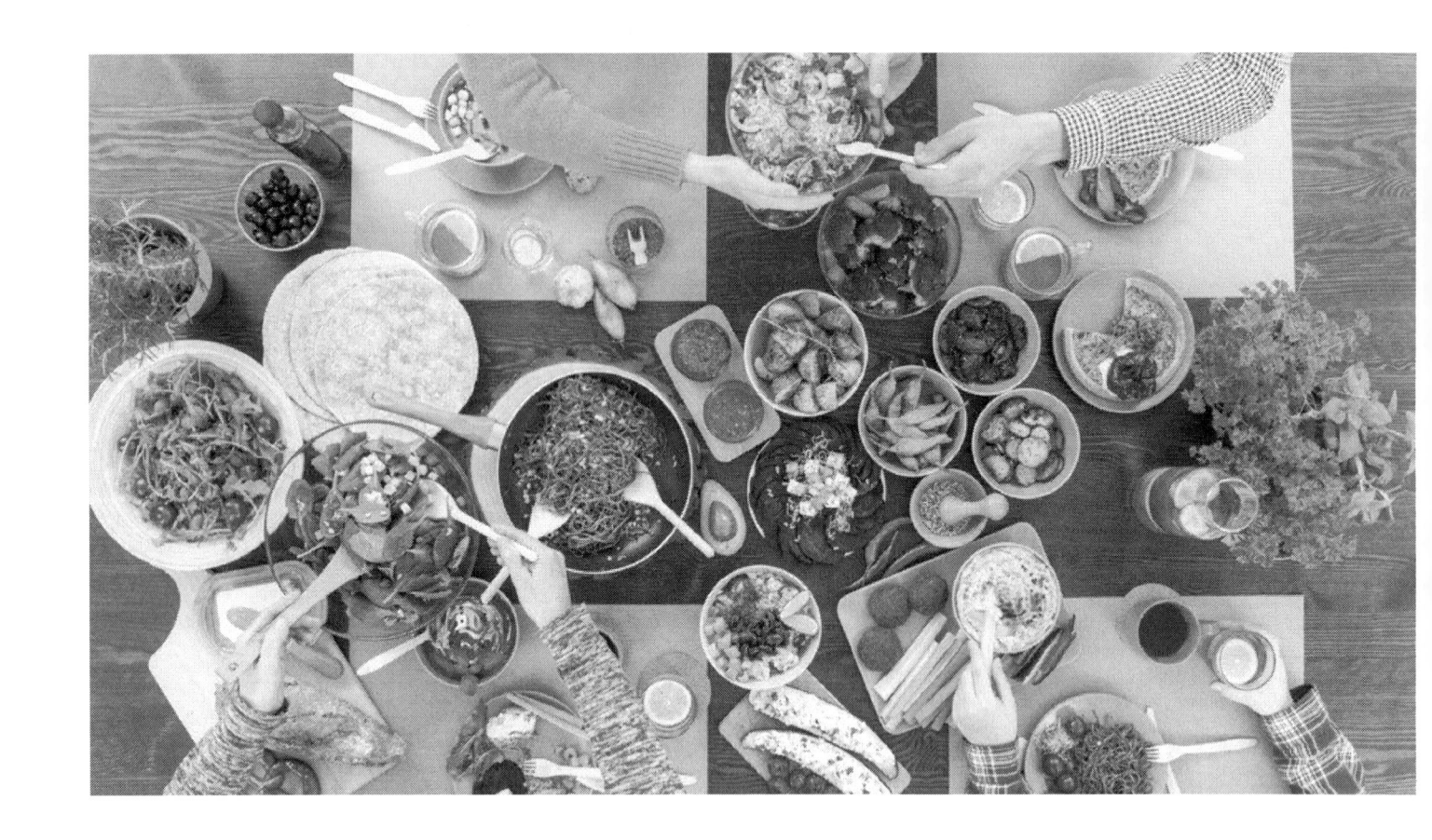

INTRODUCTION

This vegetarian-student cookbook is a useful guide for young people who are looking for tasty and simple meatless recipes. But this guide doesn't only include great recipes for vegetarians...

In chapter 1, you will find helpful information about the key vegetarian ingredients, nutritional peculiarities, suitable methods for cooking meatless meals, and the proper equipment. It can be useful for students who have just become vegetarians. The next chapter shows you a student three-week vegetarian meal plan. Check it out to be sure that you are on the right track to a healthy lifestyle.

Finally, in the last chapter, you will see more than 60 plant-based recipes that consist of common vegetarian food items. We tried to select the best recipes that include non-expensive ingredients because we realize this criterion is crucial for most college students.

All the recipes collected in the vegetarian guide are quite easy and quick, so you don't need to spend most of your precious time cooking. Using this vegetarian cookbook every student can draw up a perfect meatless menu that can satiate the stomach, increase energy levels, and boost your brain as well.

CHAPTER 1. Vegetarian Basics for College Students
Key Ingredients and Nutrients of Vegetarian Kitchen

Vegetarian eating means including fruit and veggies and excluding meat, fish, and poultry from your dietary plan. However, there are several types of vegetarianism:

- Vegans: people who don't consume meat, fish, poultry, or any animal product at all.
- Lacto-Vegetarians: people who don't consume meat, fish, or poultry, but include dairy products in their diet.
- Ovo-Vegetarians: people who consume eggs, but don't eat milk and other dairy products.
- Lacto-Ovo Vegetarians: people who don't consume meat, fish and poultry, but include dairy products, eggs, and other animal products (such as honey) in their diet.
- Semi-Vegetarians: people who sometimes consume small amounts of meat or fish.

Today more and more students arrive at the idea of becoming a vegetarian and, thus, leading a healthy lifestyle. Actually, vegetarianism of any type can offer a lot of benefits for college students.

Time Saving for Cooking
Everyone knows that vegetarian food is quite simple and quick. It isn't difficult to cook vegetarian meals and most students appreciate that. Time saving lets young people devote their spare time to more exciting or more important things.

Maintaining a Healthy Body Weight
Vegetarians usually don't have weight problems because they don't consume unhealthy fats and cholesterol as meat eaters. It's a great benefit for students who study a lot and are not very active.

Increasing Energy Levels
The vegetarian diet includes a lot of fruit and veggies as substitutes for meat, fish, and poultry filling your body with more nutrients, water and fiber that are much easier to digest. Don't forget that when your body doesn't have to work hard to digest complex foods, you will have more energy for other processes. Besides, plant-based eating is rich in oxygen which makes your body work more efficiently.

Saving Money
Students are usually on a budget. Becoming a vegetarian is a perfect way to save on your expenses. Fruit, veggies, grains, and pasta are much cheaper than meat products, fish and poultry.

Preventing Diseases
Consuming less animal fat and cholesterol can help you avoid a lot of chronic diseases, heart disease, cancer and reduce the risk of high blood pressure.

Showing Animal Compassion
If you want to make our world better, vegetarianism is what you really need. In such a way, you can demonstrate your compassionate attitude to animals and become a member of a kinder and gentler society.

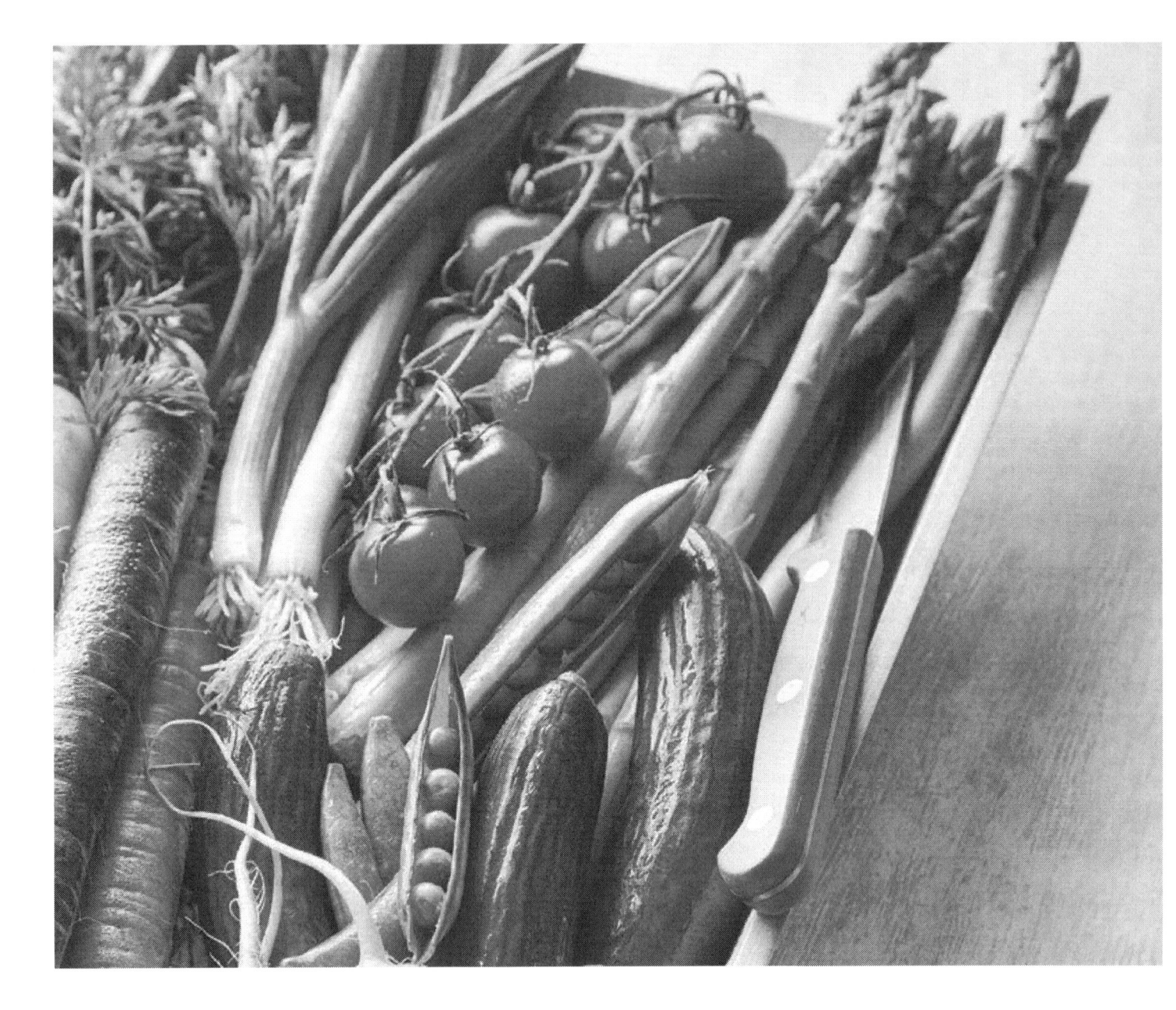

Avoiding Nutritional Deficiencies

When it comes to the vegetarian diet, you realize that it consists mostly of plant-based products. Types of vegetarian eating may vary. However, every type of vegetarianism can offer you not only health benefits but also can lead to several deficiencies. You should know about this risk and plan your plant-based diet so as to avoid any nutritional deficiencies.

Keep in mind that plant foods are also rich in nutrients and it is in your power to create a perfect nutritional vegetarian diet.

Protein
Excluding meat products doesn't mean excluding protein from your diet. Don't forget that eggs and dairy foods offer a complete protein, providing the nine crucial amino acids. Those students who prefer stricter forms of vegetarianism can get protein from soya, chia seeds, hemp seeds, beans, split peas, tofu, lentils, chickpeas, grains, nut butter, cereals, nuts, and most vegetables.

Iron
To avoid anaemia, you should be sure that you consume enough iron when eating plant-based foods. Great sources of iron include whole grains, dried fruits, iron-fortified cereals, green leafy vegetables,

seeds, beans, peas, nuts, and lentils. And one more important thing! By consuming vitamin C products, you can boost the absorption of iron (such products as citrus fruit, tomatoes, bell peppers, and dried fruit).

Vitamin B12
A deficiency in vitamin B12 can result in some physiological and nerve concerns, including megaloblastic anaemia. Most animal products (like eggs, yoghurt, cheese, etc.) can provide you vitamin B12. Plant-based food doesn't usually offer this vitamin. That's why you can obtain it with fortified products like breakfast cereals or a B12 supplement.

Zinc
Zinc deficiency can cause a lack of energy. Zinc can be found in soy and soy products, nuts, seeds, grains, dried beans, peas, lentils, tofu, bread, and fortified cereals.

Calcium
Be attentive to your bone health and consume enough calcium-rich foods. Of course, good sources of calcium are all dairy products, plant milk (such as soy or almond), tofu, fortified orange juice, almonds, sesame, tahini, and dandelion greens. Besides, you can find calcium in white beans, broccoli, nuts, and figs.

Vitamin D
Vitamin D is crucial for maintaining teeth and bone health. You can obtain this important vitamin from all dairy foods like milk, cheese, and yoghurt. Another source of Vitamin D is fleshy mushrooms.

Omega 3-Fatty Acids
To ensure efficient brain development and avoid heart disease, you need Omega 3-fatty acids. Good sources of Omega 3-fatty acids are oils, soybeans, flax seeds, walnuts, chia seeds, orange juice, and eggs.

Methods of Cooking Vegetarian Food

If you are a college student who is looking for great ways to save your time and money, meatless meals are the perfect choice for you. But you should know the best ways of cooking vegetarian food that can really satisfy you and fill you up.

Every student tries to find a balance between a delicious taste, simplicity, and healthy nutrition. How can you achieve this aim? It may sound crazy, but it's rather easy to do if you are a pure vegetarian. Here are a few secrets of cooking tasty vegetarian dishes.

Create a Balanced Meal
Try not to focus on a particular nutrient. Mix protein, fiber, fat, and carbs at meals when you want to feel fuller for longer. In chapter 3, you will find some of the best well-balanced vegetarian recipes for all types of vegetarianism. Check them out and choose the simplest ones for your student menu.

Use Slow-Roasting
Plant-based foods contain a lot of water. By using a slow-roasting menu, you can eliminate excessive liquid, intensify the flavor, and make the texture of your dish chewier.

Include Chewy Ingredients
Chewy foods such as tofu, nuts, or grilled mushrooms can make your meals more delicious and heartier. If you incorporate chewy foods, you will feel fuller and more pleasant.

Experiment with Flavor and Textures
Diversify your plate by combining various favors and textures. Creamy, crispy, chunky... Soft, spicy, sour... There is a vast selection. Don't be boring!

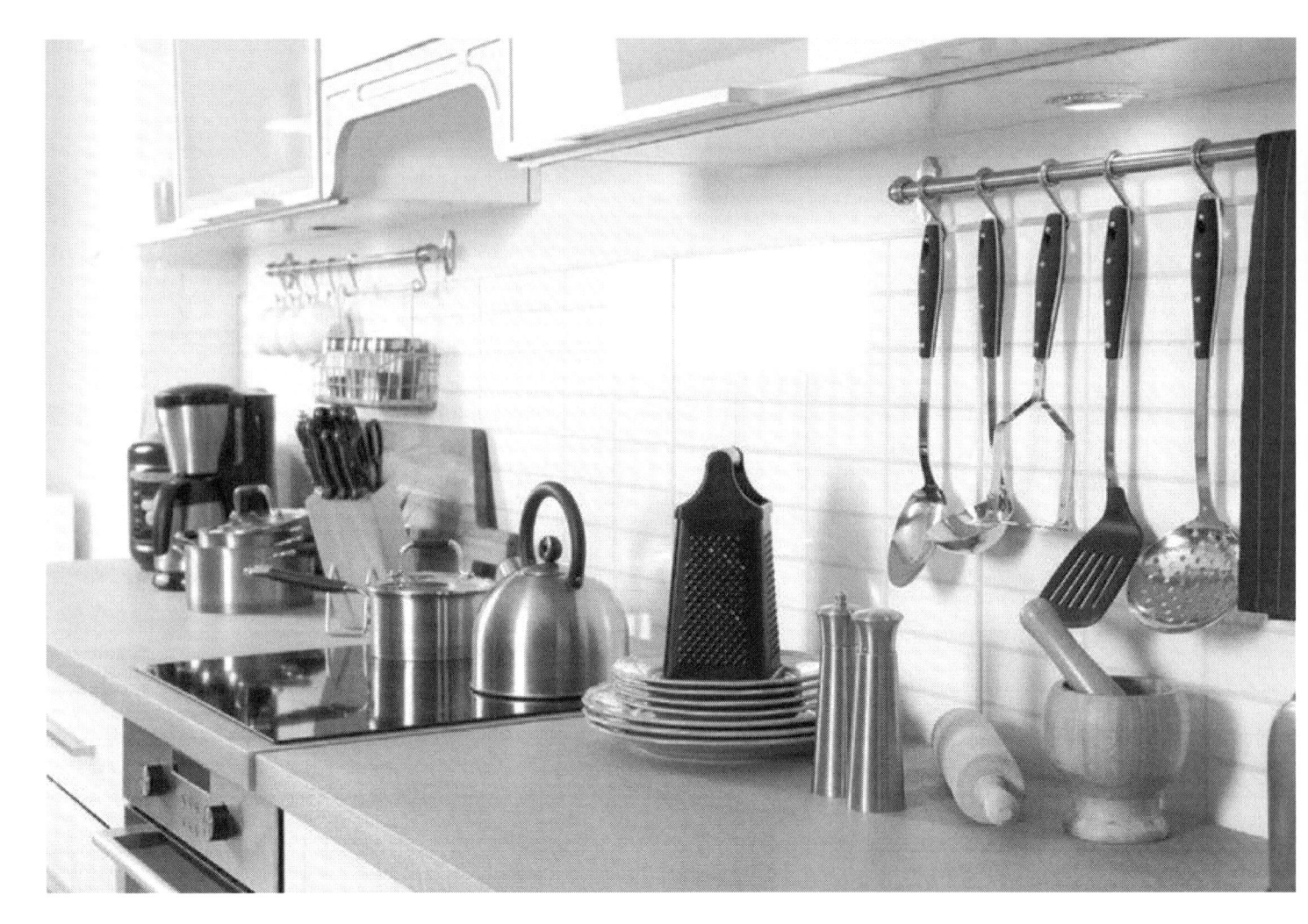

Useful Tools and Equipment

Being a college student who becomes a vegetarian means that you need to choose the right cooking equipment to help you cook your meatless meals. Don't be afraid! You don't need a lot of kitchen devices but there are some essentials without which you can't cook vegetarian dishes.

- **Blender and Food Processor**

Smoothies, hummus, pesto, salad dressings, sauces, creamy soups are meals that you can't cook without an electric blender, immersion blender or good food processor. These kitchen appliances are necessary for any vegetarian student.

- **Non-Stick Frying Pan**

To roast your ingredients, you need a pan. Try to pick out a good-quality non-stick one to make your cooking more convenient and easier.

- **Set for Stirring**

A spatula, a classic cooking spoon, and its slotted version will be your helpers in the kitchen.

- **Colander**

A vegetarian menu includes different kinds of pasta, noodles, and rice. To cook these dishes, you need a colander.

- **Knives, Grater and Can Opener**

To cut and grate your veggie ingredients, you need a good set of knives and a grater. Moreover, there are a lot of vegetarian recipes where you need to use a can opener to open canned foods.

- **Chopping Board**

Think about the place where you will cut your ingredients. Of course, it would be better to use a chopping board for this.

- **Various Saucepans**

Pots are important tools for cooking meatless meals. To boil, sauté, or simmer your vegetarian ingredients you might use different saucepans.

Making Your Vegetarian-Student Pantry

If you are a college student who switches to a vegetarian diet, you should ensure that your meatless pantry is ready to cook tasty and hearty dishes. Everyone understands that all students haven't much time and money for cooking. That is the key reason why you should think about your vegetarian menu beforehand. Here are 11 ingredients that are known as the staples for quick and delicious meatless meals.

- **Vegetables**

If you decided to become a vegetarian, you should have some veggies at home. Try to always store your favorite ones in the pantry.

- **Fresh and Dried Fruit**

To blend a smoothie in the morning or cook your favorite dessert, you need fruit. But you might not need only fresh fruit but also dried ones for some salads or even main courses.

- **Grains**

Barley, bulgar, brown and white rice, millet, etc. should be stocked in your pantry. Remember, grains can help you make your meals interesting and more nutritious.

- **Tofu**

Tofu is a cool ingredient that fits most vegetarian dishes. It is excellent for baking and frying. Look at chapter 3! Here you will find a lot of fantastic recipes with tofu.

- **Lentils**

With lots of different colors, lentils are perfect for quick meals. Quick to cook (like rice), lentils are rich in protein and have various flavors.

- **Nuts and Seeds**

One better source of protein is nuts and seeds. They should always be stored in your pantry. Most of our vegetarian recipes include various kinds of nuts and seeds.

- **Nutritional Yeast**

Nutritional yeast is a wonderful item that can add cheese flavor to your meals even if you don't put cheese into them. Besides, this ingredient can be used for cooking sauces and dips.

- **Beans**

There are so many meatless recipes with beans. Don't forget to buy frozen or canned beans to cook your favorite dishes all the time whenever you want.

- **Herbs**

To top any meal and make it more fragrant, you need herbs. It can be dill, parsley, basil, coriander, and so on.

- **Leafy Greens**

Leafy greens are perfect for fast-cooking salads, sandwiches, and snacks. Kale or spinach ingredients that can help you cook a tasty meal for lunch and dinner.

- **Oils**

To fry any food or sprinkle on any salad, you need oil. Keep olive or coconut oil in your student pantry to cook tastily and quickly.

CHAPTER 2. Three-Week Simple Vegetarian Meal Plan

Week 1

	Breakfast	**Lunch**	**Dinner**	**Dessert/Snacks**
Monday	Green Chickpea Flour Pancakes Page 16	Bell Pepper Salsa Page 28	Hearty Potato Stew Page 55	Coconut Muffins Page 68/ Potato Chips Page 32
Tuesday	Breakfast Egg Muffins Page 18	Corn Pasta with Brown Butter Page 30	Linguine with Mushrooms Page 60	Raspberry Vanilla Cream Page 67/ Greek Cheese Sandwich Page 43
Wednesday	Egg-Free French Toasts Page 19	Tri-Colored Lunch Bowl Page 24	Cold Cucumber Soup with Dill Page 53	Apple Dutch Pancake Page 63/ Bell Peppers and Hummus Page 34
Thursday	Bakes Eggs with Herbs Page 15	Avocado Toasts with Hummus Page 23	Cream Cheese Leek Risotto Page 57	Sushi with Peanut Butter and Jelly Page 62/ Warm Salad with Cauliflower Page 48
Friday	Student Tomato Omelet Page 17	Lentil Bowl with Tomato and Garlic Page 27	Chunky Chickpea Soup Page 51	Delicate Banana Pancakes Page 64/ Crispy Cheese Sticks Page 33
Saturday	Coffee Breakfast Pudding Page 20	Spicy Veggie Wraps Page 26	Indian Stew with Peanuts Page 56	Splendid Cherry Ice-Cream Page 69/ Crunchy Roasted Edamame Page 37
Sunday	High Calorie Oatmeal with Cinnamon Page 22	Buddha Mix Page 25	Broccoli Pesto Fusilli Page 58	Awesome Chocolate Mousse Page 70/ Perfect Movie Popcorn Page 35

Week 2

	Breakfast	**Lunch**	**Dinner**	**Dessert/Snacks**
Monday	Oatmeal with Almonds and Cherry Page 21	Pearl Couscous with Lemon Page 29	Moroccan Carrot Soup with Cilantro Page 52	Apple Dutch Pancake Page 63/ Perfect Movie Popcorn Page 35
Tuesday	Student Tomato Omelet Page 17	Lentil Bowl with Tomato and Garlic Page 27	Fresh Tomato Avocado Soup with Basil Page 54	Raspberry Vanilla Cream Page 67/ Bell Peppers and Hummus Page 34
Wednesday	Coffee Breakfast Pudding Page 20	Spicy Veggie Wraps Page 26	Noodles with Carrot and Sesame Page 59	Splendid Cherry Ice-Cream Page 69/ Crunchy Roasted Edamame Page 37
Thursday	Baked Eggs with Herbs Page 15	Buddha Mix Page 25	Marinated Tofu with Peanuts Page 61	Sushi with Peanut Butter and Jelly Page 62/ Warm Salad with Cauliflower Page 48
Friday	Egg-Free French Toasts Page 19	Bell Pepper Salsa Page 28	Cream Cheese Leek Risotto Page 57	Coconut Muffins Page 68/ Potato Chips Page 32
Saturday	Breakfast Egg Muffins Page 18	Tri-Colored Lunch Bowl Page 24	Cold Cucumber Soup with Dill Page 53	Raspberry Vanilla Cream Page 67/ California Sandwich with Veggies Page 42
Sunday	Green Chickpea Flour Pancakes Page 16	Avocado Toasts with Hummus Page 23	Linguine with Mushrooms Page 60	Strawberry Cheesecake Toast Page 66/ Sandwich with Egg Salad Page 42

Week 3

	Breakfast	**Lunch**	**Dinner**	**Dessert/Snacks**
Monday	High Calorie Oatmeal with Cinnamon Page 22	Buddha Mix Page 25	Marinated Tofu with Peanuts Page 61	Delicate Banana Pancakes Page 64/ Greek Cheese Sandwich Page 43
Tuesday	Coffee Breakfast Pudding Page 20	Tri-Colored Lunch Bowl Page 24	Broccoli Pesto Fusilli Page 58	Raspberry Vanilla Cream Page 67/ California Sandwich with Veggies Page 40
Wednesday	Student Tomato Omelet Page 17	Bell Pepper Salsa Page 28	Indian Stew with Peanuts Page 56	Coconut Muffins Page 68/ Toasted Pumpkin Seeds Page 38
Thursday	Oatmeal with Almonds and Cherry Page 21	Corn Pasta with Brown Butter Page 30	Fresh Tomato Avocado Soup with Basil Page 54	Splendid Cherry Ice-Cream Page 69/ Low-Calorie Kale Chips Page 36
Friday	Egg-Free French Toasts Page 19	Spicy Veggie Wraps Page 26	Hearty Potato Stew Page 55	Apple Dutch Pancake Page 63/ Perfect Movie Popcorn Page 35
Saturday	Bakes Eggs with Herbs Page 15	Avocado Toasts with Hummus Page 23	Moroccan Carrot Soup with Cilantro Page 52	Strawberry Cheesecake Toast Page 66/ Sandwich with Egg Salad Page 42
Sunday	Green Chickpea Flour Pancakes Page 16	Pearl Couscous with Lemon Page 29	Chunky Chickpea Soup Page 51	Awesome Chocolate Mousse Page 70/ Potato Chips Page 32

CHAPTER 3. Easy and Healthy Vegetarian Recipes for College Students

BREAKFAST

Baked Eggs with Herbs

Prep time: 5 minutes

Cooking time: 10 minutes

Servings: 2

Nutrients per serving:

Carbohydrates – 3 g

Fat – 54 g

Protein – 19 g

Calories – 579

Ingredients:

- 4 eggs
- 100g baby spinach, chopped
- 1 cup double cream
- 4 Tbsp fresh pesto
- 1 Tbsp cheese, grated
- Salt and pepper, to taste

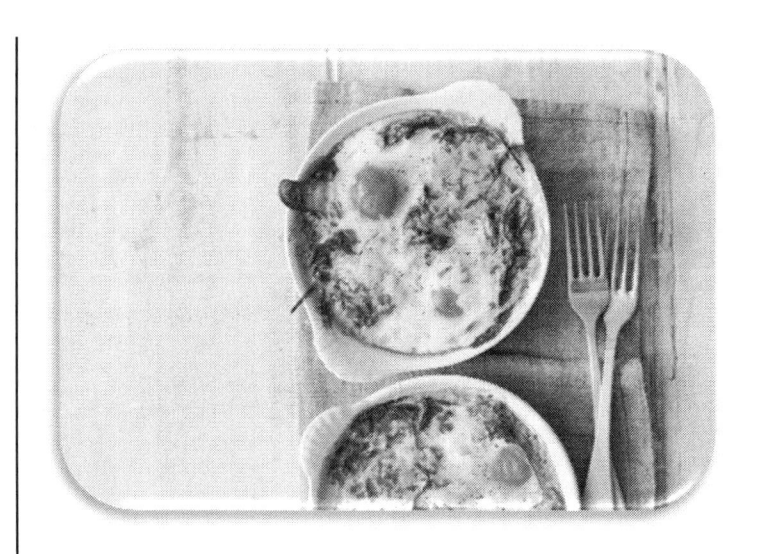

Instructions:

1. Blend the pesto, spinach, cream, salt and pepper. Divide this mixture into 2 separate dishes. Top both with the cheese.
2. Make two hollows in each dish and break an egg into each hollow.
3. Place in the oven (preheated up to 180°C) and cook for 10 minutes.

Green Chickpea Flour Pancakes

Prep time: 5 minutes

Cooking time: 5 minutes

Servings: 4

Nutrients per serving:

Carbohydrates – 33.8 g

Fat – 10.1 g

Protein – 10.1 g

Calories – 253

Ingredients:

- 1 cup chickpea flour
- 1 cup water
- 3 spring onions, chopped
- ½ tsp salt
- ½ tsp pepper
- 1 tsp turmeric
- 1 Tbsp olive oil

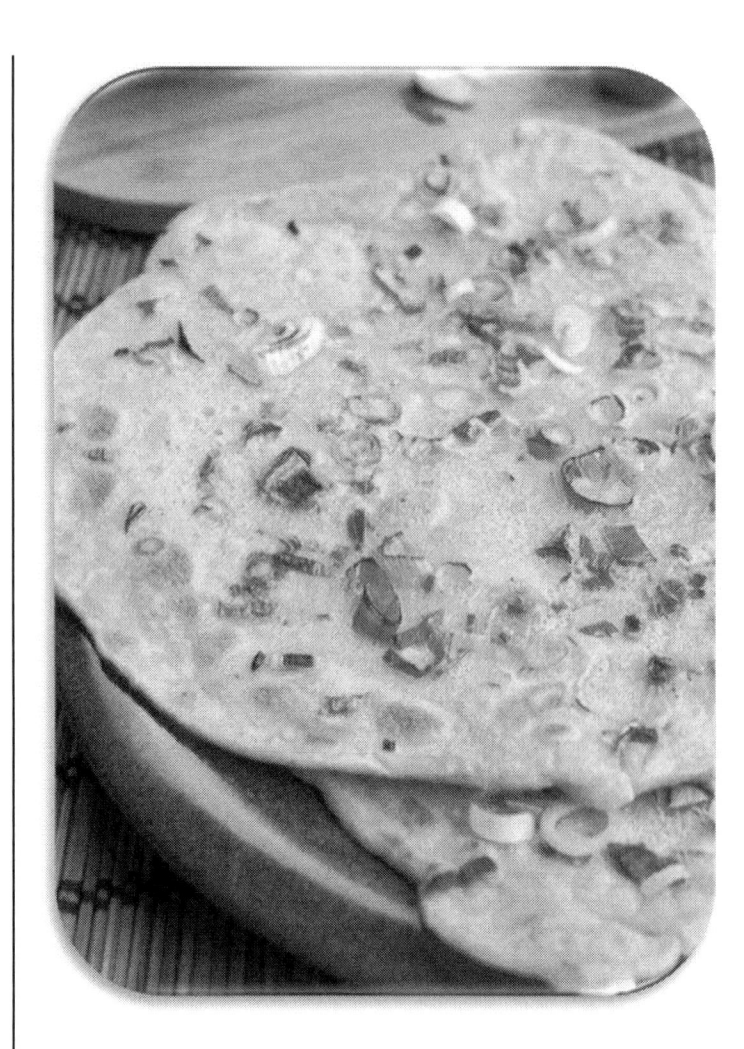

Instructions:

1. Using a blender, mix the water, chickpea flour, turmeric, salt, and pepper. Add the chopped onions and heat the oil in the pan.
2. Pour the chickpea mixture into the pan and cook for 3 minutes.

Student Tomato Omelet

Prep time: 2 minutes

Cooking time: 8 minutes

Servings: 1

Nutrients per serving:

Carbohydrates – 11.2 g

Fat – 25.3 g

Protein – 20.2g

Calories – 342

Ingredients:

- 2 eggs
- 2 Tbsp olive oil
- ½ cup cherry tomatoes, chopped
- ½ cup basil, fresh or dried
- ¼ cup favorite cheese, grated
- Salt and pepper, to taste

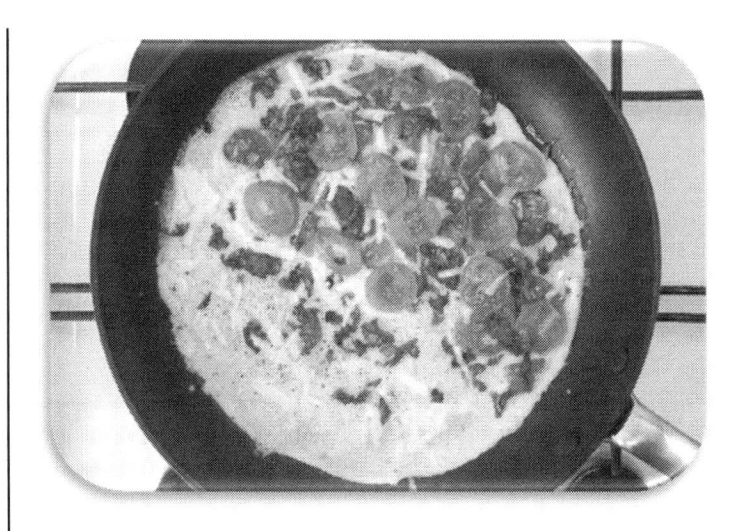

Instructions:

1. Heat 1 Tbsp oil on the pan and cook the chopped tomatoes for 2 minutes. Put them aside.
2. Put the beaten eggs in a separate bowl. Add salt and pepper. Whisk well.
3. Heat the remaining oil in the pan and put the egg mixture in it. Fry it for about 2 minutes. Then add the tomatoes, basil, and cheese.

Breakfast Egg Muffins

Prep time: 5 minutes

Cooking time: 20 minutes

Servings: 3

Nutrients per serving:

Carbohydrates – 4 g

Fat – 15 g

Protein – 17 g

Calories – 219

Ingredients:

- 1 red bell pepper, diced
- 2 spring onions, diced
- 6 eggs
- 1 handful spinach, washed and chopped
- ½ cup Cheddar cheese, grated
- 1 tsp salt
- 1 tsp curry powder
- 2 Tbsp olive oil

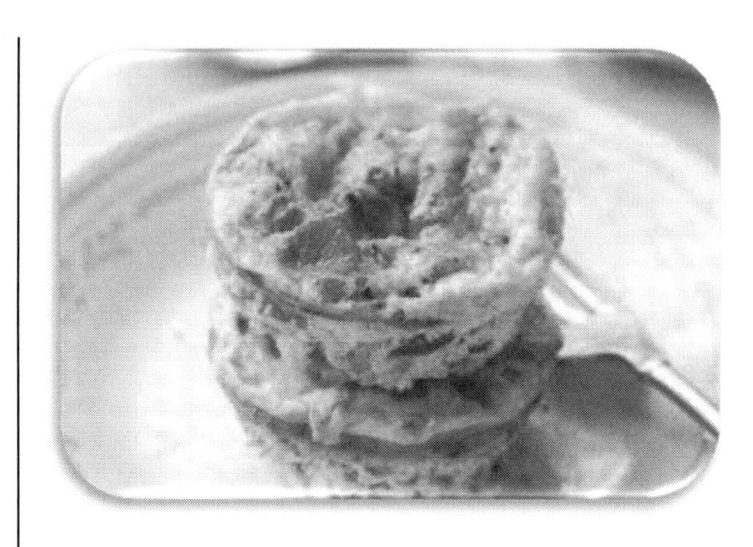

Instructions:

1. In a bowl mix the diced bell pepper and onions. Add the chopped spinach, eggs and salt and stir thoroughly.
2. Put the cheese and curry powder into the bowl and whisk.
3. Sprinkle the muffin tin with oil and put the egg mixture into the muffin slots.
4. Place your muffins in the oven (preheated up to 200°C) and cook for 20 minutes.

Egg-Free French Toast

Prep time: 5 minutes

Cooking time: 10 minutes

Servings: 6

Nutrients per serving:

Carbohydrates – 12.7 g

Fat – 12.7 g

Protein – 2.9 g

Calories – 145

Ingredients:

- 1 cup almond milk
- 2 Tbsp all-purpose flour
- 2 Tbsp nutritional yeast
- 2 Tbsp butter, melted
- 2 tbsp brown sugar
- 1 tsp cinnamon
- ½ tsp vanilla extract
- 1 pinch salt
- 6 slices bread

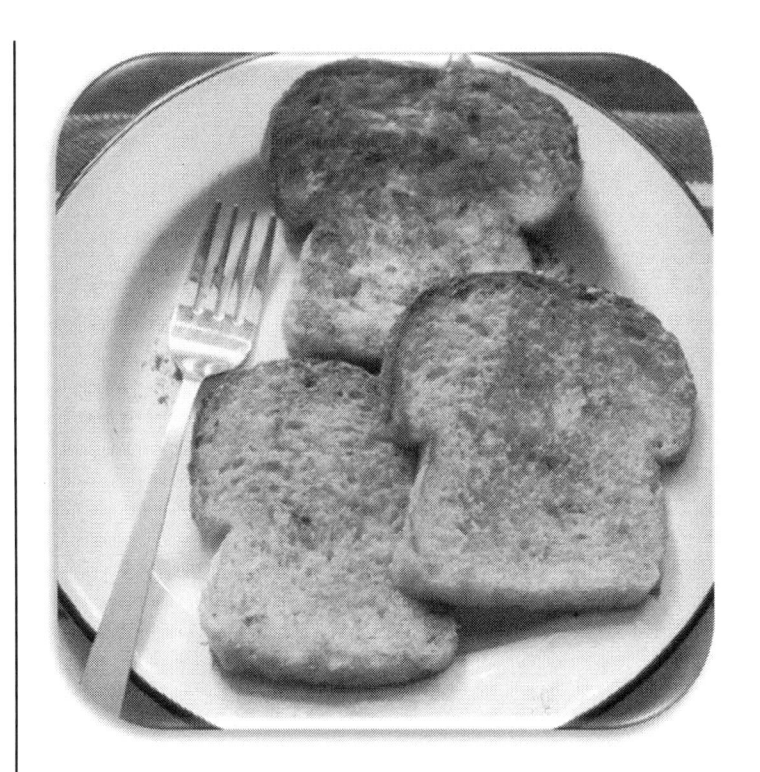

Instructions:

1. In a separate bowl, blend the almond milk, flour, nutritional yeast, brown sugar, cinnamon, vanilla extract, and salt. Dunk each bread slice into this mixture.
2. Place the butter in the pan and add your bread slices. Cook for about 2 minutes on each side until brown.

Coffee Breakfast Pudding

Prep time: 3 minutes

Cooking time: 3 minutes

Servings: 2

Nutrients per serving:

Carbohydrates – 12.6 g

Fat – 24 g

Protein – 5.9 g

Calories – 282

Ingredients:

- 4 Tbsp chia seeds
- 1 cup coffee, brewed and cooled
- 1 cup coconut milk
- 1 Tbsp almond butter
- 1 tsp vanilla paste
- 2 Tbsp erythritol
- ½ tsp cinnamon

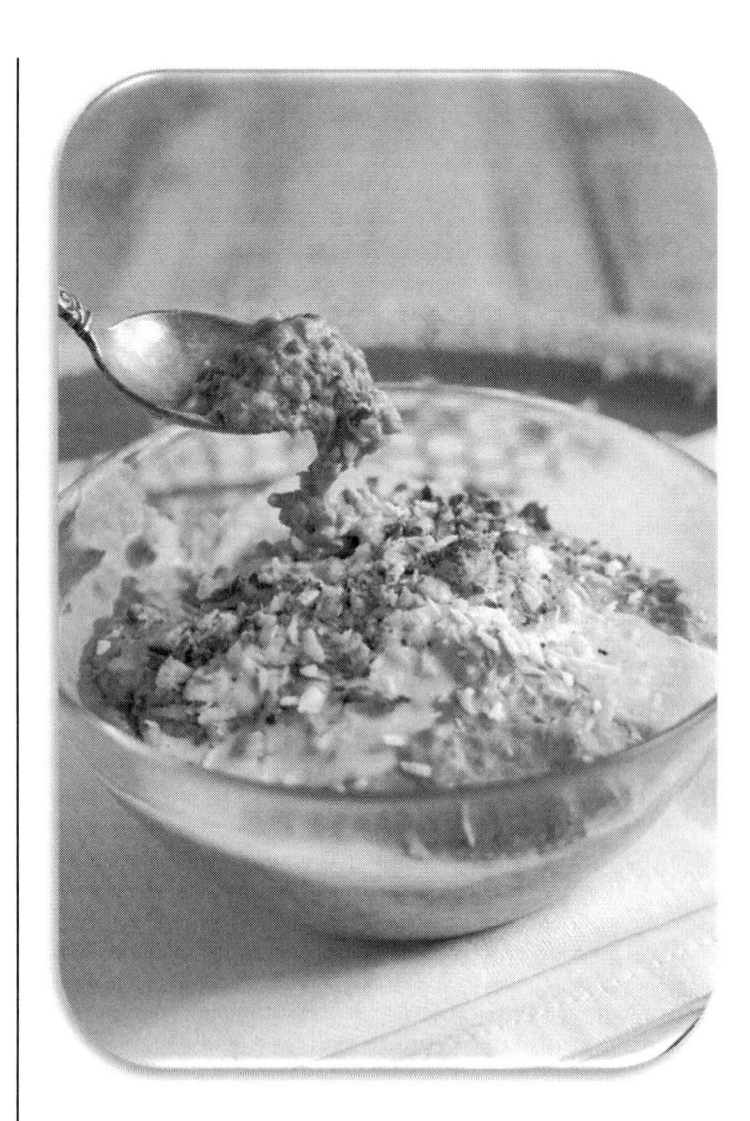

Instructions:

1. Combine all the pudding ingredients in a separate bowl and stir thoroughly.
2. Cover and put in the fridge overnight.

Oatmeal with Almonds and Cherry

Prep time: 5 minutes

Cooking time: 10 minutes

Servings: 2

Nutrients per serving:

Carbohydrates – 37 g

Fat – 13 g

Protein – 10 g

Calories – 300

Ingredients:

- 2 Tbsp almonds, sliced and toasted
- ½ cup old fashioned rolled oats
- 1 cup vanilla almond milk, unsweetened
- ½ tsp almond extract
- ¼ cup cherries, fresh

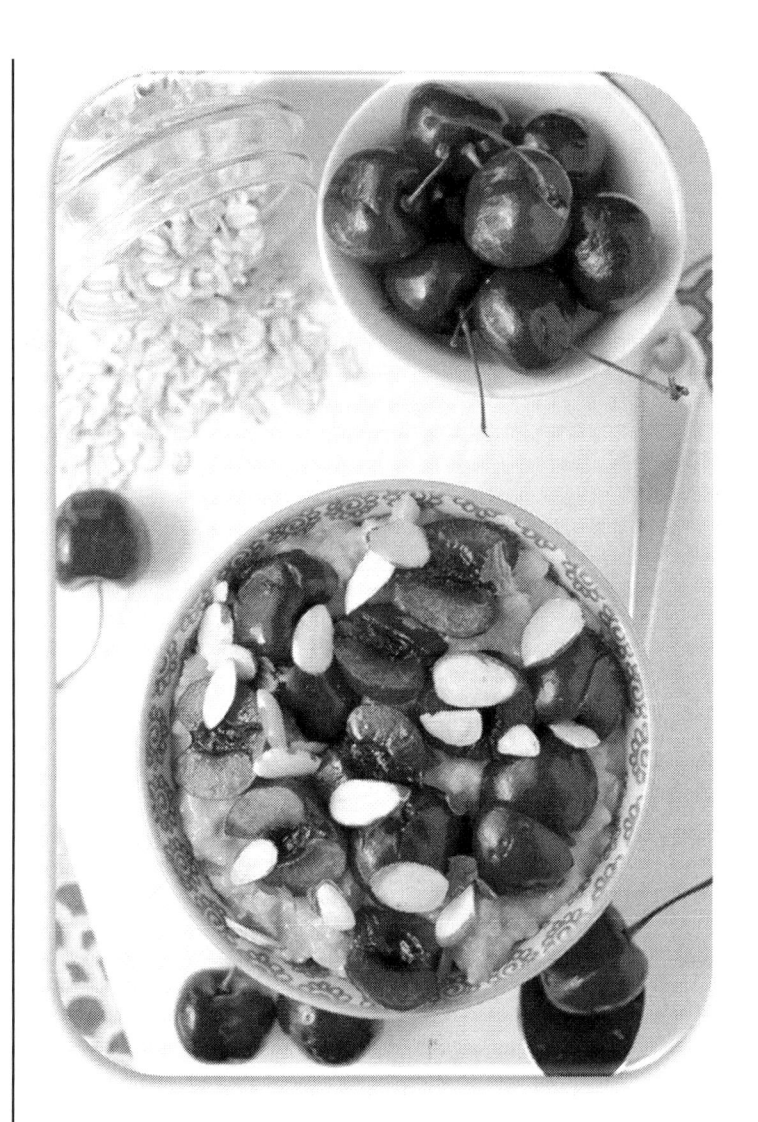

Instructions:

1. Pour the almond milk in a saucepan and boil. Add the oats and cook for 5 minutes.
2. Sprinkle the oats with almond extract. Top it with cherries and sliced almonds.

High Calorie Oatmeal with Cinnamon

Prep time: 5 minutes

Cooking time: 5 minutes

Servings: 1

Nutrients per serving:

Carbohydrates – 50 g

Fat – 24 g

Protein – 13 g

Calories – 452

Ingredients:

- ½ cup rolled oats
- 1 Tbsp apricots, dried and sliced
- 1 Tbsp coconut flakes
- 1 Tbsp sunflower seeds
- 2 tbsp almonds, chopped
- ½ tsp cinnamon
- 1 cup almond milk

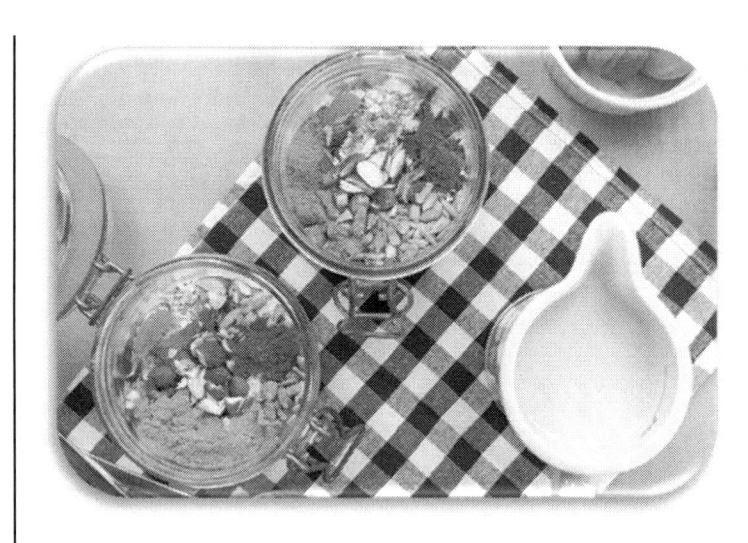

Instructions:

1. Place all the ingredients for your vegetarian oatmeal in a separate bowl and mix thoroughly. Pour in the almond milk and enjoy your breakfast!

LUNCH

Avocado Toasts with Hummus

Prep time: 5 minutes

Cooking time: 0 minutes

Servings: 1

Nutrients per serving:

Carbohydrates – 50 g

Fat – 23 g

Protein – 18 g

Calories – 462

Ingredients

- 2 slices bread
- 2 Tbsp garlic hummus
- ½ avocado, sliced
- 3 slices red onion
- 2 Tbsp hemp seeds
- Cilantro for decoration

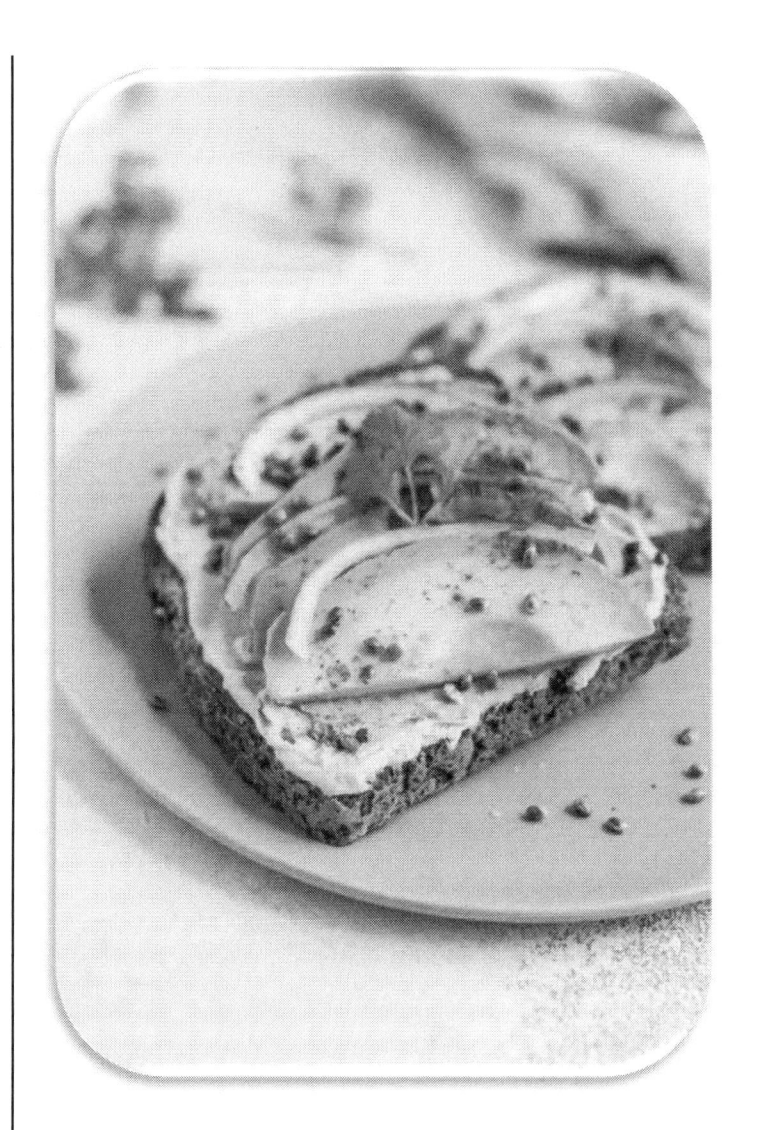

Instructions:

1. Spread 1 Tbsp hummus on each bread slice.
2. Put the sliced avocado, red onion and hemp seeds on each bread slice.
3. Top with cilantro.

Tri-Colored Lunch Bowl

Prep time: 20 minutes

Cooking time: 10 minutes

Servings: 4

Nutrients per serving:

Carbohydrates – 46 g

Fat – 3 g

Protein – 13 g

Calories – 424

Ingredients:

- 1-pound box tri-colored pasta
- 1 handful baby kale, chopped
- 1 handful spinach, chopped
- 2 cups yellow cherry tomatoes, sliced
- ¼ cup fresh basil, chopped
- ½ cup white wine vinegar
- 3 Tbsp lemon juice
- 1 tsp extra virgin olive oil
- 1 tsp dried Italian seasoning
- ½ tsp ground sea salt
- Ground black pepper, to taste

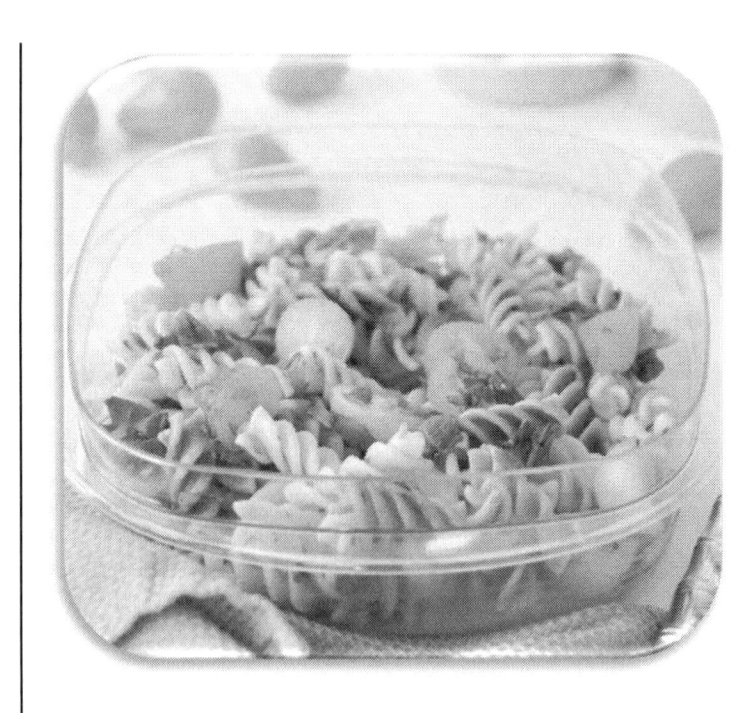

Instructions:

1. Put the vinegar, olive oil, lemon juice, salt, Italian seasoning, and black pepper into a bowl. Whisk well.
2. Read the instructions on the package and cook the pasta. Blend the pasta with chopped greens and tomatoes.
3. Sprinkle the pasta mixture with the dressing and stir thoroughly.

Buddha Mix

Prep time: 10 minutes

Cooking time: 20 minutes

Servings: 2

Nutrients per serving:

Carbohydrates – 90 g

Fat – 22 g

Protein – 22 g

Calories – 600

Ingredients:

- ½ cup uncooked grains (rice, barley, millet, etc.)
- 3 cups leafy greens (spinach, kale, cabbage, broccoli, bell pepper, etc.)
- 1 cup cooked legumes (any beans, chickpeas, peas, edamame, etc.)

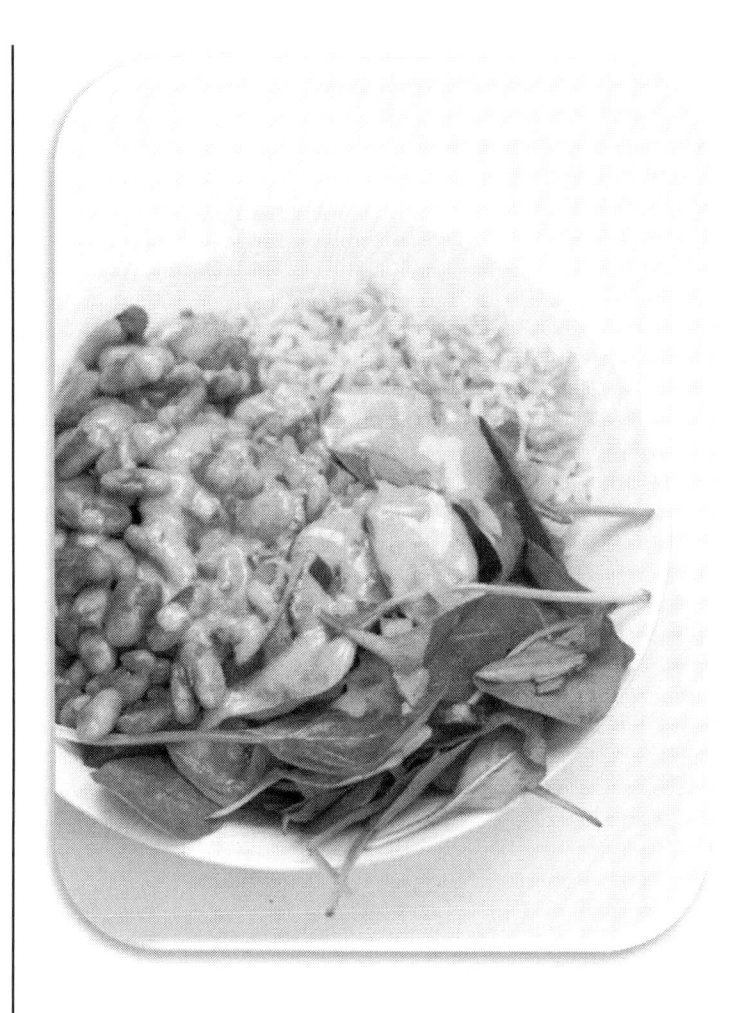

Instructions:

1. Cook your grains.
2. Chop the greens.
3. Make a tasty dressing.
4. Combine all your ingredients and mix them thoroughly.

Spicy Veggie Wrap

Prep time: 25 minutes

Cooking time: 0 minutes

Servings: 2

Nutrients per serving:

Carbohydrates – 41 g

Fat – 15 g

Protein – 14 g

Calories – 342

Ingredients:

- 2 carrots, grated
- 3 Tbsp sunflower seeds, roasted
- 1 red onion, chopped
- ¼ red bell pepper, diced
- 1 handful spinach, washed, drained and chopped
- 1 thumb ginger, grated
- ¼ cup cottage cheese
- 2 Tbsp sour cream
- 1 tsp lemon zest
- 3 tsp mustard
- 2 wraps
- Salt and pepper, to taste

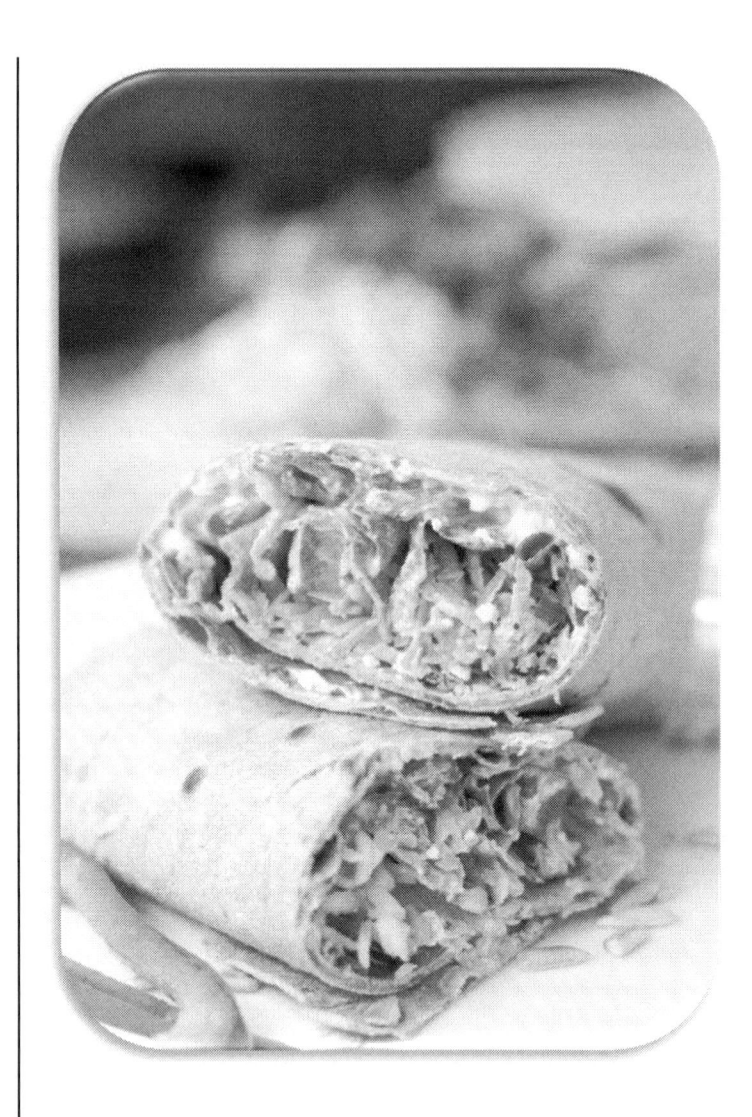

Instructions:

1. Mix the cottage cheese, ginger, lemon zest, mustard and sour cream in a bowl. Stir thoroughly.
2. Spread the dressing on the wrap and layer the bell peppers, carrots and onions on it. Top the veggies with the roasted sunflower seeds. Add salt and pepper.
3. Roll the veggie wrap and serve.

Lentil Bowl with Tomatoes and Garlic

Prep time: 5 minutes

Cooking time: 25 minutes

Servings: 6

Nutrients per serving:

Carbohydrates – 49 g

Fat – 3 g

Protein – 21 g

Calories – 294

Ingredients:

- 1 Tbsp olive oil
- 2 onions, finely chopped
- 4 cloves garlic, minced
- 2 cups brown lentils, dried and rinsed
- 1 tsp salt
- ½ tsp ground ginger
- ½ tsp paprika
- 3 cups water
- ¼ tsp pepper
- ¼ cup lemon juice
- 3 Tbsp tomato paste
- ½ tomato, chopped
- 1 cup fat-free plain Greek yoghurt

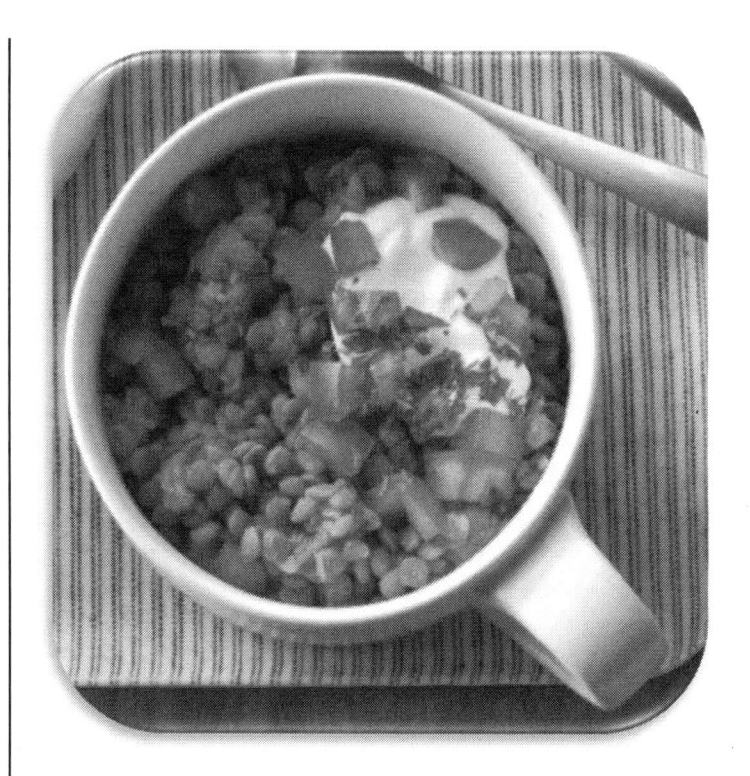

Instructions:

1. Using a big saucepan sauté the onions for 2 minutes. Put in the garlic and cook for 1 minute more. Add the lentils, seasoning and water. Simmer for 25 minutes.
2. Put lemon juice and tomato paste in the saucepan.
3. Top with the chopped tomatoes and greens.
4. Serve with yoghurt.

Bell Pepper Salsa

Prep time: 10 minutes

Cooking time: 10 minutes

Servings: 4

Nutrients per serving:

Carbohydrates – 15 g

Fat – 116 g

Protein – 3 g

Calories – 206

Ingredients:

- 1 green pepper, diced
- 1 red pepper, diced
- 1 yellow pepper, diced
- 4 garlic cloves, peeled
- ¼ cup lime juice
- 3 jalapeños, seedless
- 1 red onion, peeled and chopped
- ½ cup fresh cilantro, minced
- 1 tsp kosher salt

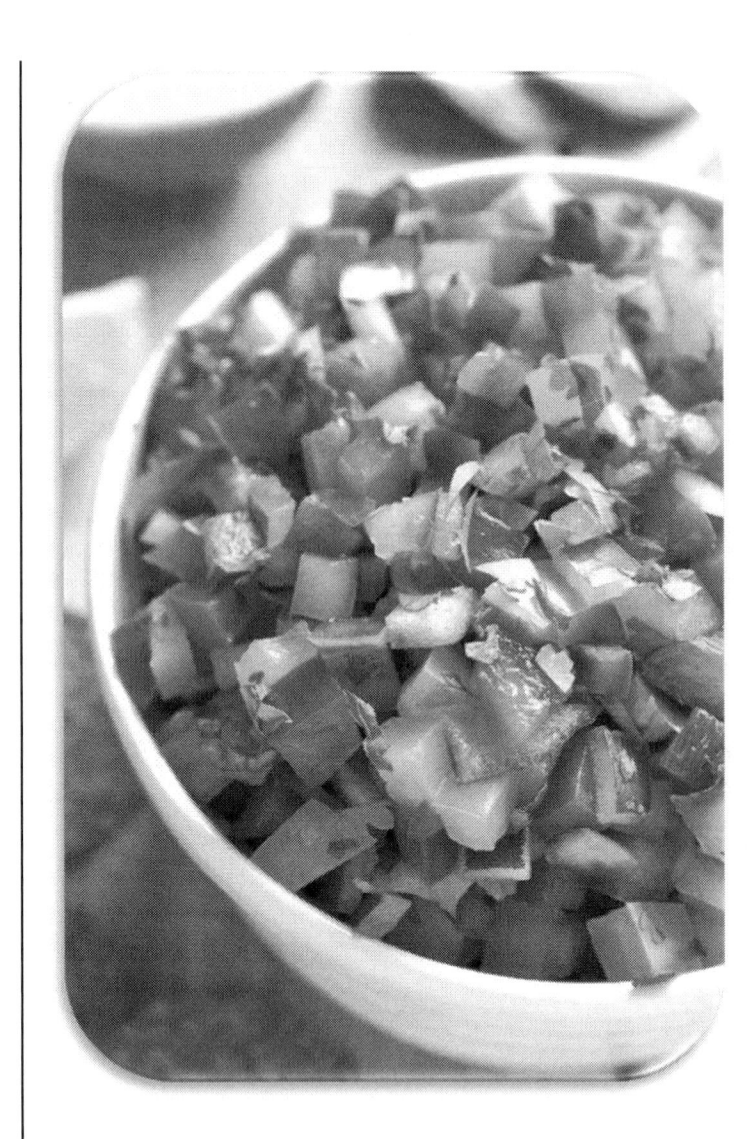

Instructions:

1. Combine all the ingredients except for the cilantro.
2. Garnish with cilantro.

Pearl Couscous with Lemon

Prep time: 10 minutes

Cooking time: 5 minutes

Servings: 4

Nutrients per serving:

Carbohydrates – 32.2 g

Fat – 7.2 g

Protein – 7 g

Calories – 225

Ingredients:

- 1¼ cups water
- 1 cup pearl couscous
- 1 tsp kosher salt
- 1 Tbsp olive oil
- 1 cup scallions, sliced
- 1 clove garlic
- 1 tsp lemon zest
- 1 cup peas
- ¼ tsp pepper

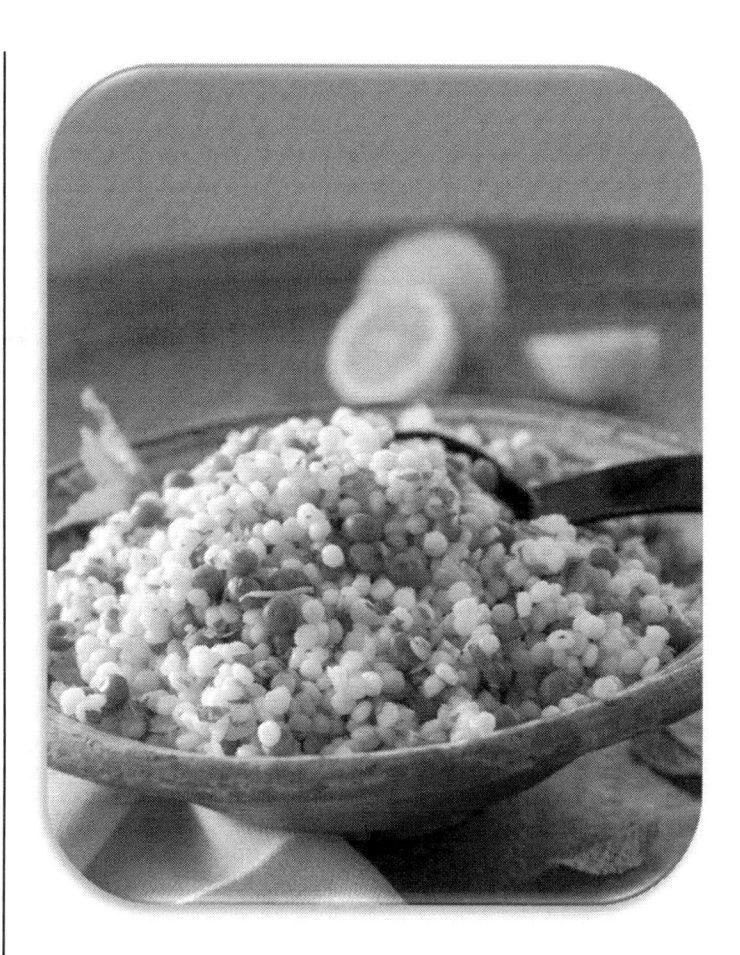

Instructions:

1. Cook the couscous for about 9 minutes. Don't forget to add ½ tsp salt when cooking.
2. Sauté the scallions for 4-5 minutes. Add the garlic and cook for 1 minute more. Add the lemon zest.
3. Combine the scallion mixture and peas with couscous in a bowl. Stir well.
4. Add the remaining salt and pepper.

Corn Pasta with Brown Butter

Prep time: 5 minutes

Cooking time: 10 minutes

Servings: 6

Nutrients per serving:

Carbohydrates – 18.2 g

Fat – 40.4 g

Protein – 14 g

Calories – 495

Ingredients:

- 2 cups sweet corn kernels
- 1 cup campanelle pasta
- 6 Tbsp butter
- 1 cup Parmesan cheese, grated
- ¼ cup packed fresh basil leaves
- Salt and pepper, to taste

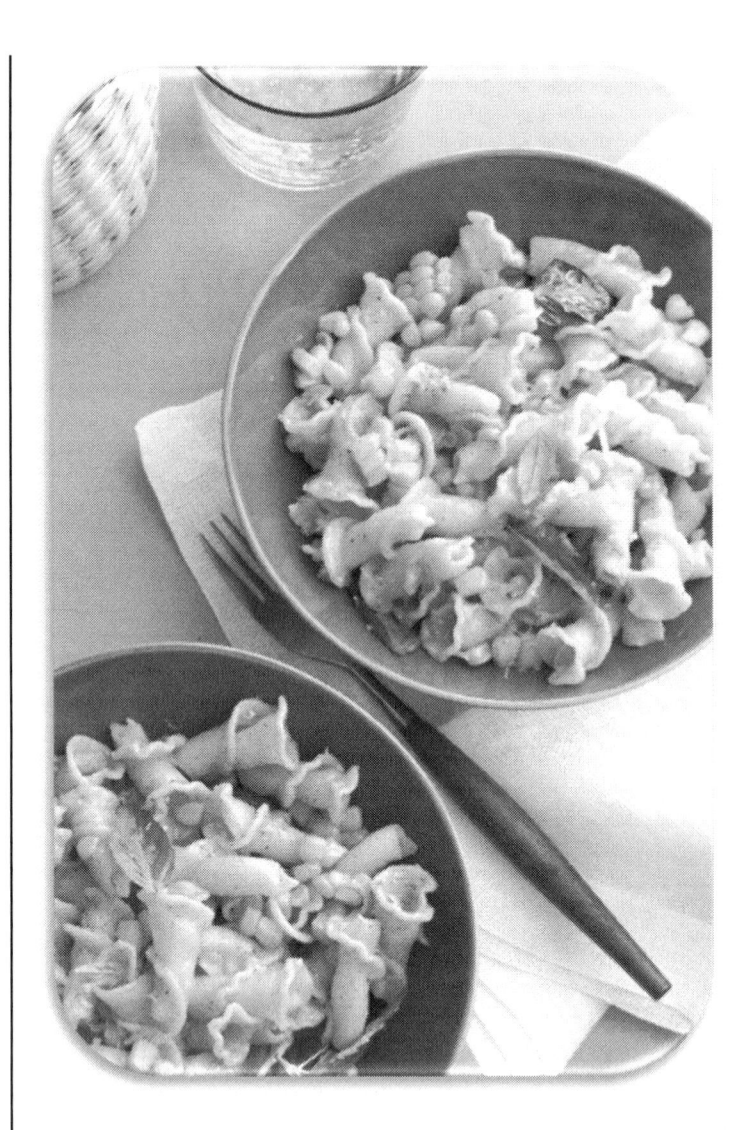

Instructions:

1. Cook the pasta. Drain it and put it aside.
2. In a saucepan, melt the butter and cook it for about 2-4 minutes. Add the corn and ¼ tsp salt and pepper. Cook for 2 minutes and then set aside.
3. Combine the pasta with the corn mixture. Add basil, parmesan, and salt. Stir thoroughly.

SNACKS & QUICK BITES

Simple Garlic Bread Snack

Prep time: 10 minutes

Cooking time: 10 minutes

Servings: 2

Nutrients per serving:

Carbohydrates – 38 g

Fat – 45 g

Protein – 9 g

Calories –596

Ingredients:

- 1 long baguette-style bread
- ¼ cup butter, softened
- 3 cloves garlic, minced
- 1 Tbsp fresh parsley, chopped
- ½ cup Parmesan cheese, grated
- Salt and pepper, to taste

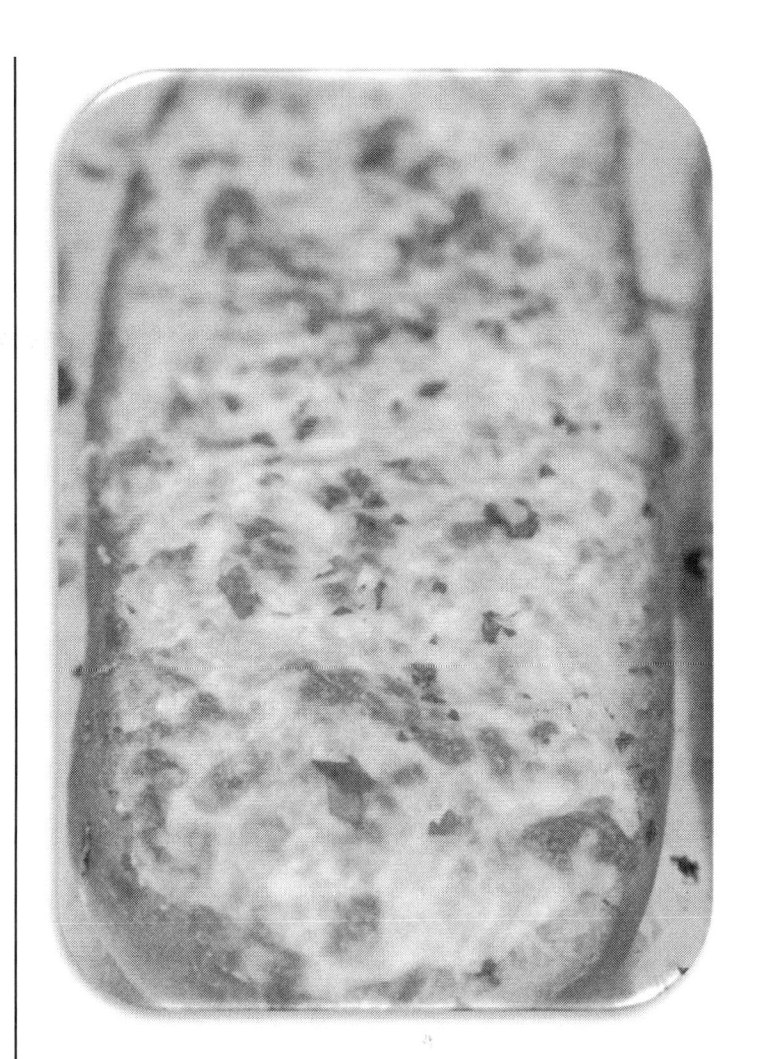

Instructions:

1. In a separate bowl, blend the butter, minced garlic, parmesan cheese, and parsley.
2. Split your bread in half and spread the butter mix over each piece.
3. Put in the preheated oven at 190°C.
4. Bake for 10 minutes.

Potato Chips

Prep time: 10 minutes

Cooking time: 30 minutes

Servings: 4

Nutrients per serving:

Carbohydrates – 19 g

Fat – 7 g

Protein – 2 g

Calories – 143

Ingredients:

- 4 potatoes, finely sliced
- 3 Tbsp olive oil
- Vegetable-oil cooking spray
- Salt & pepper, to taste

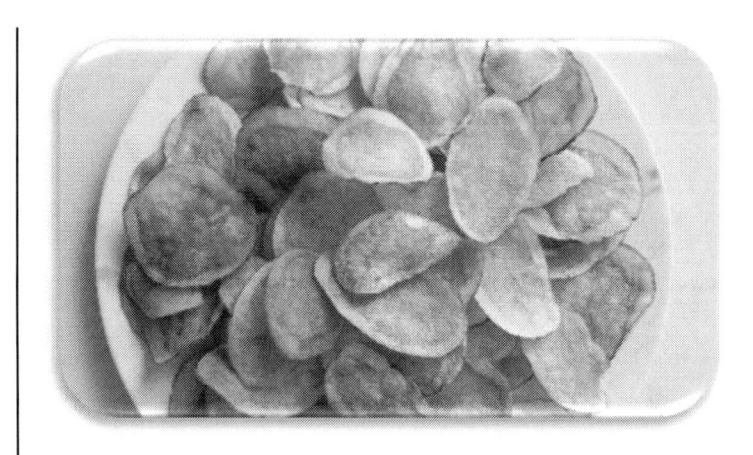

Instructions:

1. Put the potato slices in a bowl. Sprinkle them with olive oil. Add salt and pepper. Mix thoroughly.
2. Cover your baking sheet with cooking spray and place the potato slices on it.
3. Put your potato slices in the oven already preheated to 190°C.
4. Bake for about 30 minutes.

Crispy Cheese Sticks

Prep time: 15 minutes

Cooking time: 15 minutes

Servings: 8

Nutrients per serving:

Carbohydrates – 29.5 g

Fat – 22.5 g

Protein – 19.4 g

Calories – 400

Ingredients:

- ¼ cup water
- 2 eggs, beaten
- ½ tsp garlic salt
- 1½ cups Italian seasoned bread crumbs
- ⅓ cup corn-starch
- ⅔ cup all-purpose flour
- 2 Tbsp olive oil
- 16 ounces Mozzarella cheese sticks

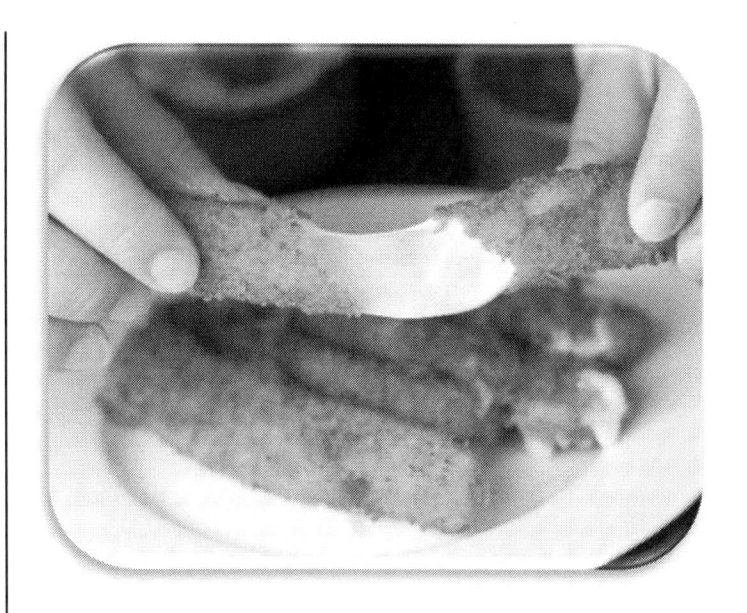

Instructions:

1. In a separate bowl, blend the water and the beaten eggs.
2. In another bowl, mix the breadcrumbs and garlic salt.
3. Mix the flour and corn-starch in a separate bowl and stir thoroughly.
4. Place each Mozzarella stick on the flour mix, then on the egg mix and finally on the bread crumbs.
5. Put your Mozzarella sticks in the frying pan. Cook about 30 seconds on each side.

Bell Peppers and Hummus

Prep time: 25 minutes

Cooking time: 10 minutes

Servings: 2

Nutrients per serving:

Carbohydrates – 44.1 g

Fat – 26.9 g

Protein – 15.9 g

Calories – 445

Ingredients:

- ½ cup red bell peppers, roasted
- ⅓ cup lemon juice
- ¼ tsp basil, chopped
- 2 cloves garlic, minced
- 1 can garbanzo beans, drained
- ⅓ cup tahini
- Salt and pepper, to taste

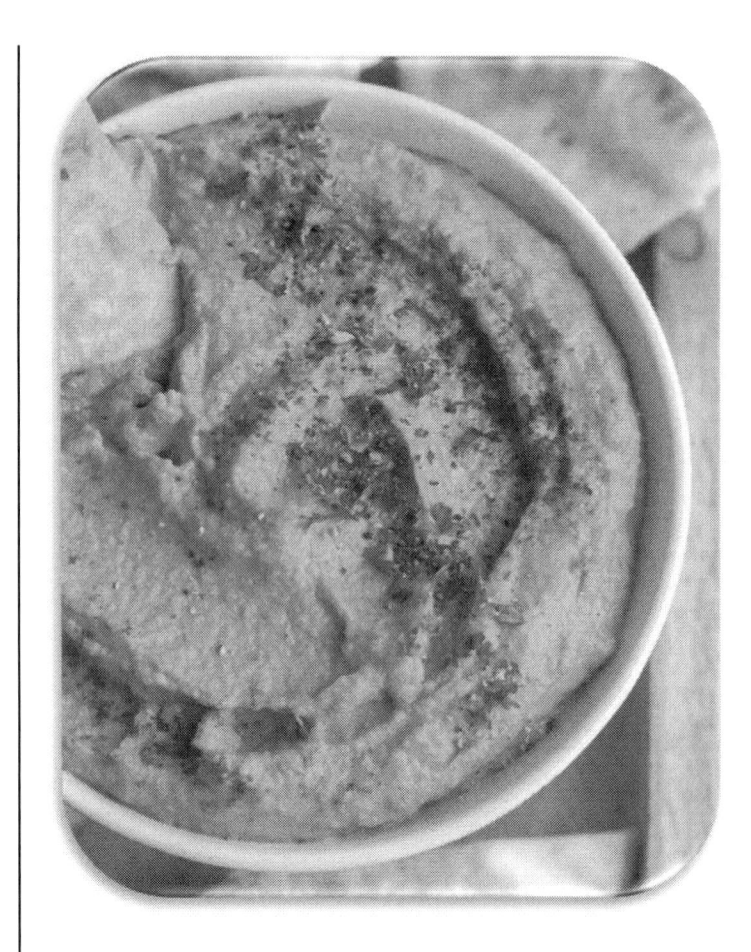

Instructions:

1. Using an electric food processor, mix the garlic, garbanzo beans, tahini and lemon juice. Blend until smooth. Add roasted peppers and continue processing for about 30 seconds.
2. Add salt and pepper.
3. Cover with chopped basil and serve.

Perfect Movie Popcorn

Prep time: 1 minute

Cooking time: 5 minutes

Servings: 3

Nutrients per serving:

Carbohydrates – 21 g

Fat – 2.1 g

Protein – 3.1 g

Calories – 120

Ingredients:

- ½ cup popcorn kernels
- 2 Tbsp avocado oil
- 1 Tbsp butter
- Salt, to taste

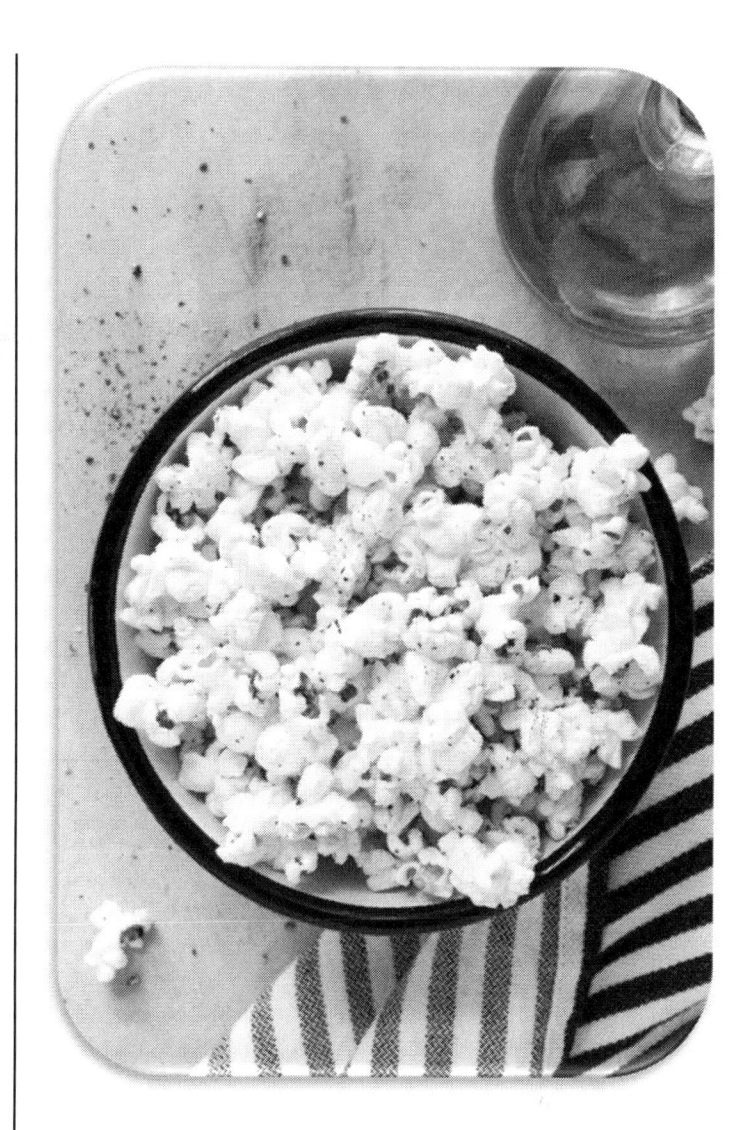

Instructions:

1. Spoon the avocado oil into the pot and heat it.
2. Put 2-3 popcorn kernels into the pot and wait for them to pop.
3. Take the pot off the stove, add the remaining kernels to the oil and wait for 1 minute.
4. Bring the pot back and cook your popcorn for 1-2 minutes.

Low-Calorie Kale Chips

Prep time: 10 minutes

Cooking time: 10 minutes

Servings: 6

Nutrients per serving:

Carbohydrates – 7.6 g

Fat – 2.8 g

Protein – 2.5 g

Calories – 58

Ingredients:

- 1 bundle kale, washed, dried and torn into bite pieces
- 1 Tbsp olive oil
- 1 tsp seasoned salt

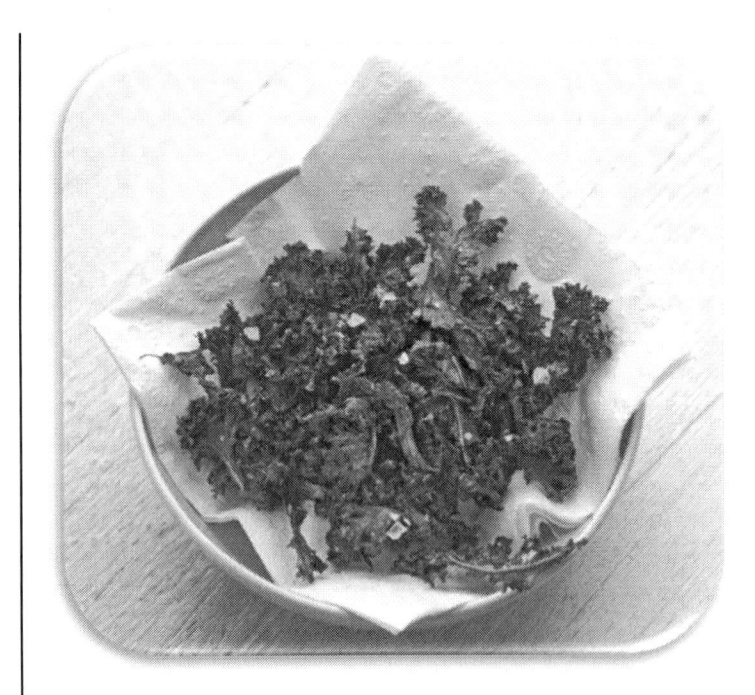

Instructions:

1. Sprinkle your kale with olive oil and seasoning salt.
2. Put the kale pieces in the oven preheated to 175°C and bake for about 10 minutes.

Crunchy Roasted Edamame

Prep time: 5 minutes

Cooking time: 20 minutes

Servings: 6

Nutrients per serving:

Carbohydrates – 6.7 g

Fat – 8.4 g

Protein – 7.4 g

Calories – 126

Ingredients:

- 1 package edamame, frozen in their pods
- 2 Tbsp extra-virgin olive oil
- 2 cloves garlic, minced
- 1 tsp sea salt
- ½ tsp ground black pepper

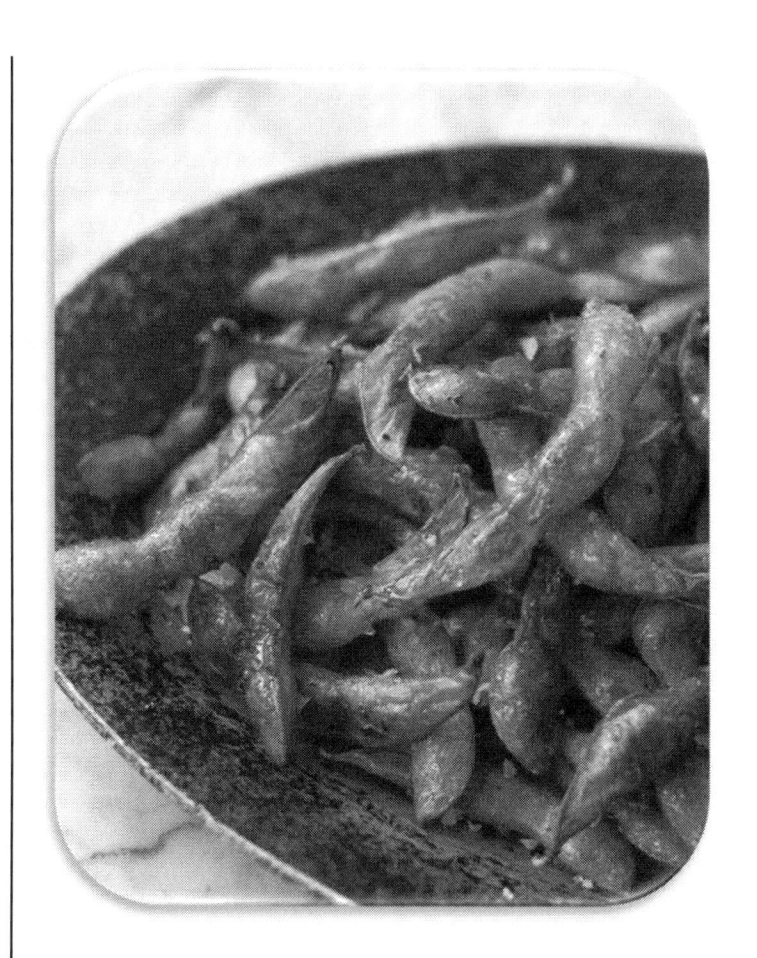

Instructions:

1. In a separate bowl, drizzle the edamame with sea salt, black pepper, and olive oil. Stir thoroughly and spread on a baking sheet.
2. Cook in the oven preheated to 190°C oven for about 20 minutes.

Toasted Pumpkin Seeds

Prep time: 10 minutes

Cooking time: 25 minutes

Servings: 6

Nutrients per serving:

Carbohydrates – 2 g

Fat – 9 g

Protein – 5 g

Calories – 105

Ingredients:

- 1½ cups pumpkin seeds
- 2 tsp butter, melted
- 1 pinch salt

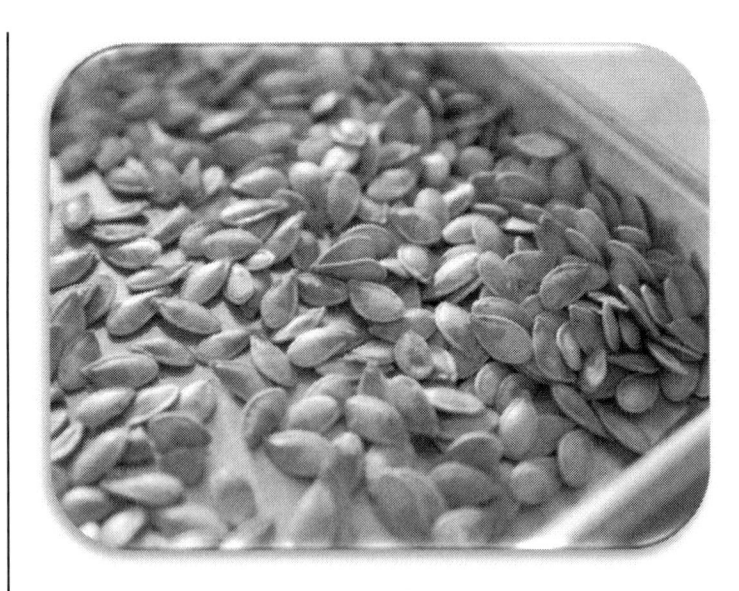

Instructions:

1. Stir the pumpkin seeds, melted butter and salt together.
2. Spread the pumpkin seeds on a baking sheet. Keep on stirring until they are golden brown. Cook for about 25 minutes.

Almond Oat No-Bake Energy Balls

Prep time: 10 minutes

Cooking time: 20 minutes

Servings: 24

Nutrients per serving:

Carbohydrates – 21 g

Fat – 6 g

Protein – 5 g

Calories – 148

Ingredients:

- 2½ cups rolled oats
- ½ cup pumpkin seeds, raw pepitas
- ½ cup raisins
- 2 Tbsp sunflower seeds, raw
- 1 tsp cinnamon
- ½ cup almond butter
- ½ cup honey
- 2 Tbsp barley malt syrup
- 1 tsp vanilla extract

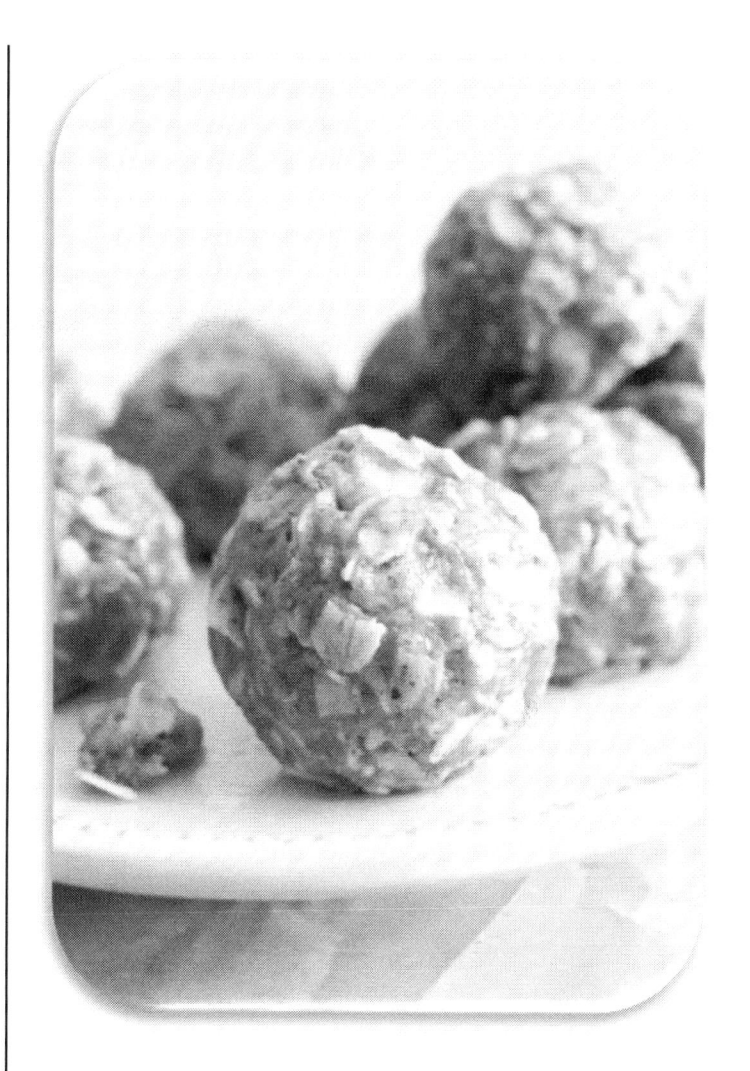

Instructions:

1. Using a blender, make the powder from ½ cup oats and ¼ cup pumpkin seeds. Put aside.
2. Blend the remaining oats, pumpkin seeds, sunflower seeds, raisin, and cinnamon in a separate bowl. Add the almond butter, barley malt syrup, honey, and vanilla extract. Stir thoroughly to get a dough consistency.
3. Create small balls from your dough and coat each one in the oat-pumpkin powder. Put in a freezer for 20 minutes.

SANDWICHES, SALADS & DRESSINGS

California Sandwich with Grilled Veggies

Prep time: 30 minutes

Cooking time: 20 minutes

Servings: 2

Nutrients per serving:

Carbohydrates – 36.5 g

Fat – 23.8 g

Protein – 9.2 g

Calories – 393

Ingredients:

- ¼ cup mayonnaise
- 3 cloves garlic, minced
- 1 Tbsp lemon juice
- ⅛ cup olive oil
- 1 cup red bell pepper, sliced
- 1 zucchini, sliced
- 1 red onion, sliced
- 1 yellow squash, sliced
- 1 loaf of bread, cut horizontally
- ½ cup feta cheese, crumbled

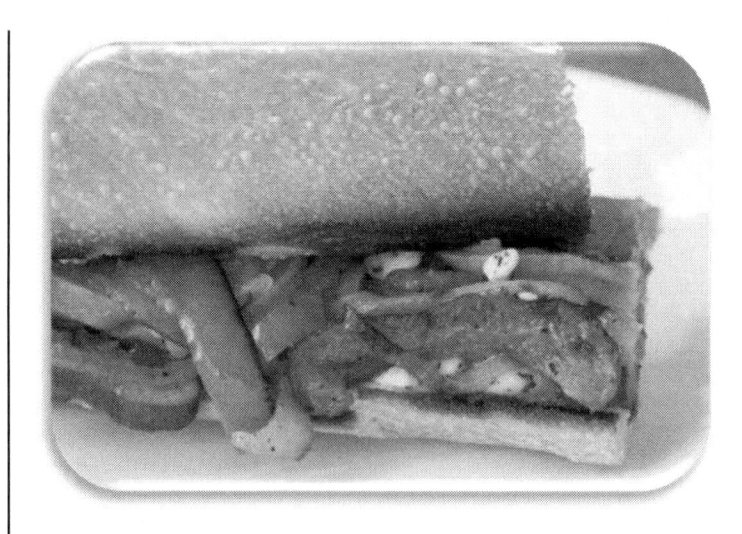

Instructions:

1. Blend the minced garlic, mayonnaise and lemon juice in a separate bowl. Put this mix aside in the fridge.
2. Sprinkle your vegetables with olive oil on each side and grill them for about 3 minutes on each side.
3. Take the mayonnaise mix and spread it on the cut sides of the bread. Add crumbled feta cheese and put the bread under the grill for 2-3 minutes.
4. Add your grilled veggies and enjoy your tasty sandwich.

Grilled Cheese Sandwich

Prep time: 5 minutes

Cooking time: 15 minutes

Servings: 2

Nutrients per serving:

Carbohydrates – 25.7 g

Fat – 28.3 g

Protein – 11.1 g

Calories –400

Ingredients:

- 4 slices white bread
- 5 Tbsp butter, softened and divided
- 2 slices Cheddar cheese

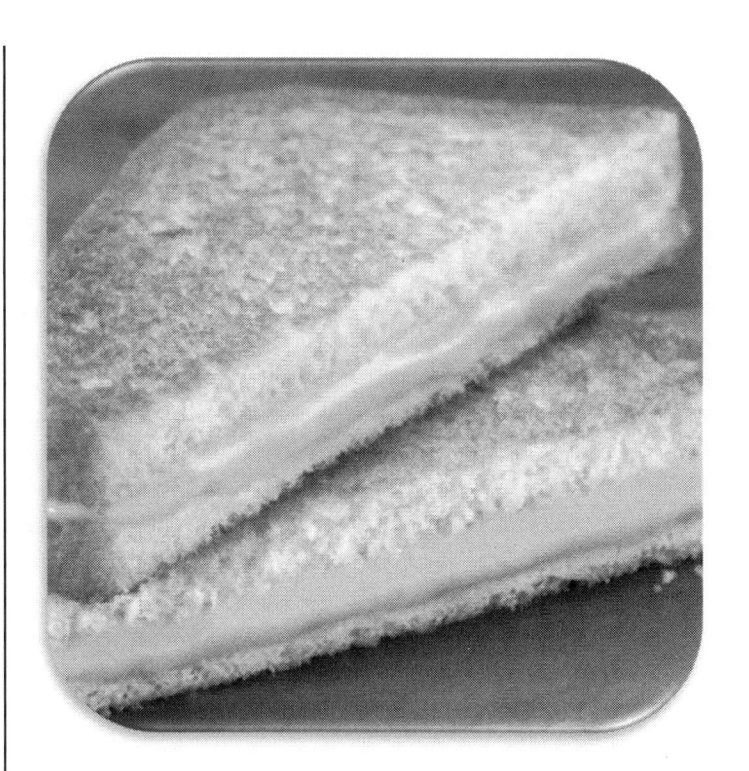

Instructions:

1. Put 1 Tbsp butter in a skillet and heat it.
2. Get two buttered bread slices and put them butter side down on the skillet.
3. Cover the two slices of bread with cheese and top them with the remaining bread. Grill until they are lightly brown and the cheese is melted.

Sandwich with Egg Salad

Prep time: 10 minutes

Cooking time: 20 minutes

Servings: 4

Nutrients per serving:

Carbohydrates – 25 g

Fat – 17 g

Protein – 17 g

Calories –315

Ingredients:

- 6 hard-boiled eggs, peeled and chopped
- 3 Tbsp mayonnaise
- 2 tsp Dijon mustard
- ¼ cup green onions, chopped
- 8 slices whole wheat bread
- 4 lettuce leaves
- Salt and pepper, to taste
- Garlic powder, to taste

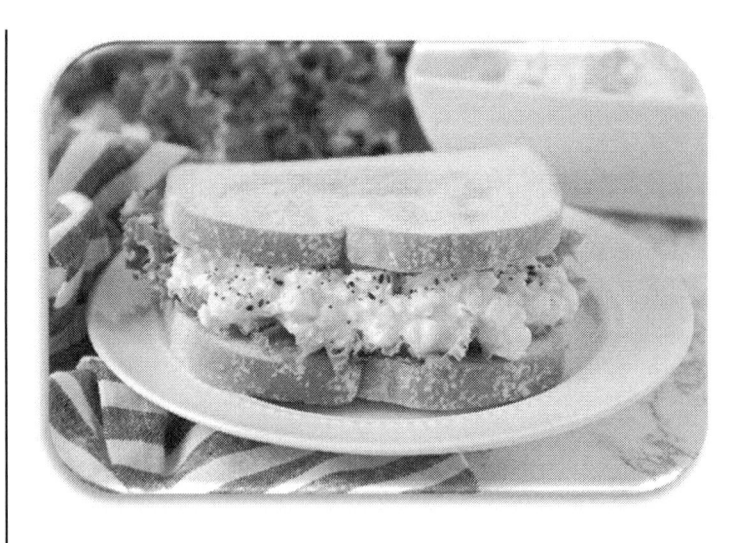

Instructions:

1. In a separate bowl, mix the chopped eggs, onion, mustard, garlic powder, mayonnaise, salt, and pepper. Stir thoroughly.
2. Put a lettuce leaf and spread ½ cup of egg salad on a slice of bread. Cover it with another slice of bread.

Greek Cheese Sandwich

Prep time: 5 minutes

Cooking time: 5 minutes

Servings: 1

Nutrients per serving:

Carbohydrates – 27.1 g

Fat – 30.9 g

Protein – 24.6 g

Calories –482

Ingredients:

- 1½ tsp butter, softened
- 2 slices whole wheat bread
- 2 Tbsp Feta cheese, crumbled
- 2 slices Cheddar cheese
- 1 Tbsp red onion, chopped
- ¼ tomato, sliced

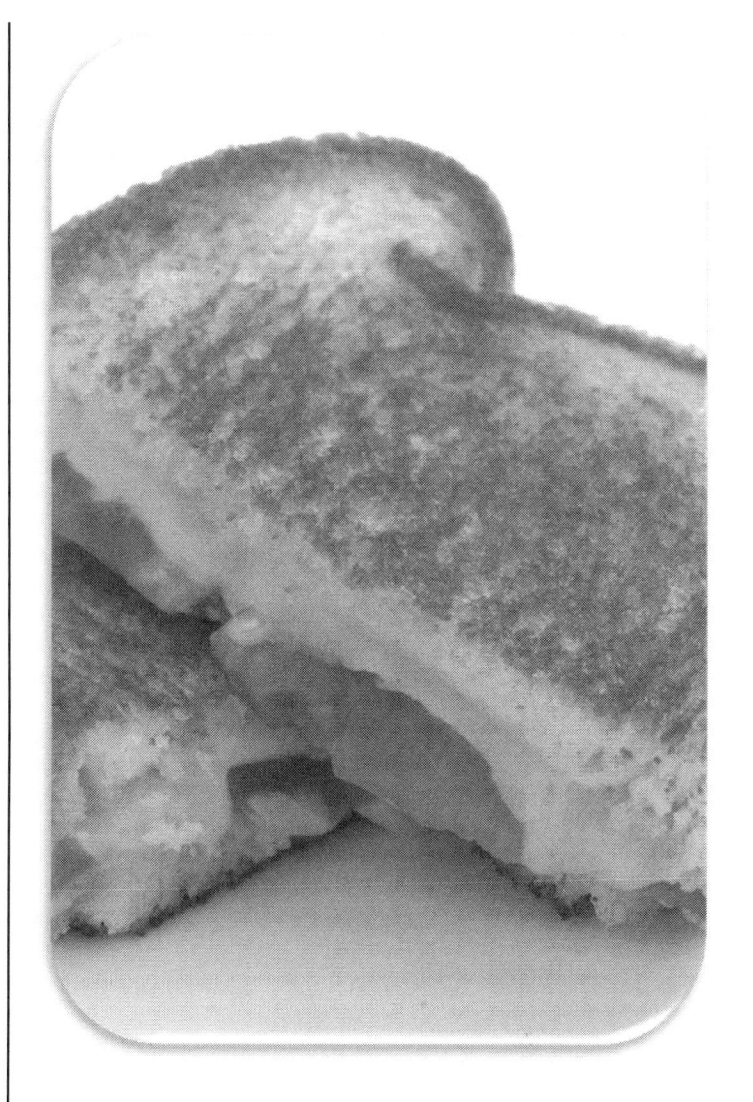

Instructions:

1. Take a non-buttered bread slice and layer Feta cheese, Cheddar cheese, tomato slices, and red onion on it.
2. Get one slice of buttered bread and put it on the layered slice of bread.
3. Fry your sandwich for about 2 minutes on each side until it is golden brown.

Wild Rice Salad with Pomegranate, Pistachio and Persimmon

Prep time: 5 minutes

Cooking time: 5 minutes

Servings: 4

Nutrients per serving:

Carbohydrates – 24.3 g

Fat – 12.5 g

Protein – 17.1 g

Calories – 208

Ingredients:

- 1 cup pomegranate seeds
- 3 cups wild rice, cooked
- 2 tsp honey
- 1 Tbsp extra-virgin olive oil
- 1 Tbsp white wine vinegar
- 2 Tbsp red miso paste
- ¼ cup orange juice
- 1 shallot, chopped and soaked in ice water
- 4 Fuyu persimmons, trimmed and diced
- 1 cup pistachios, roasted, salted and chopped
- 4 ounces kale
- Salt and ground black pepper, to taste

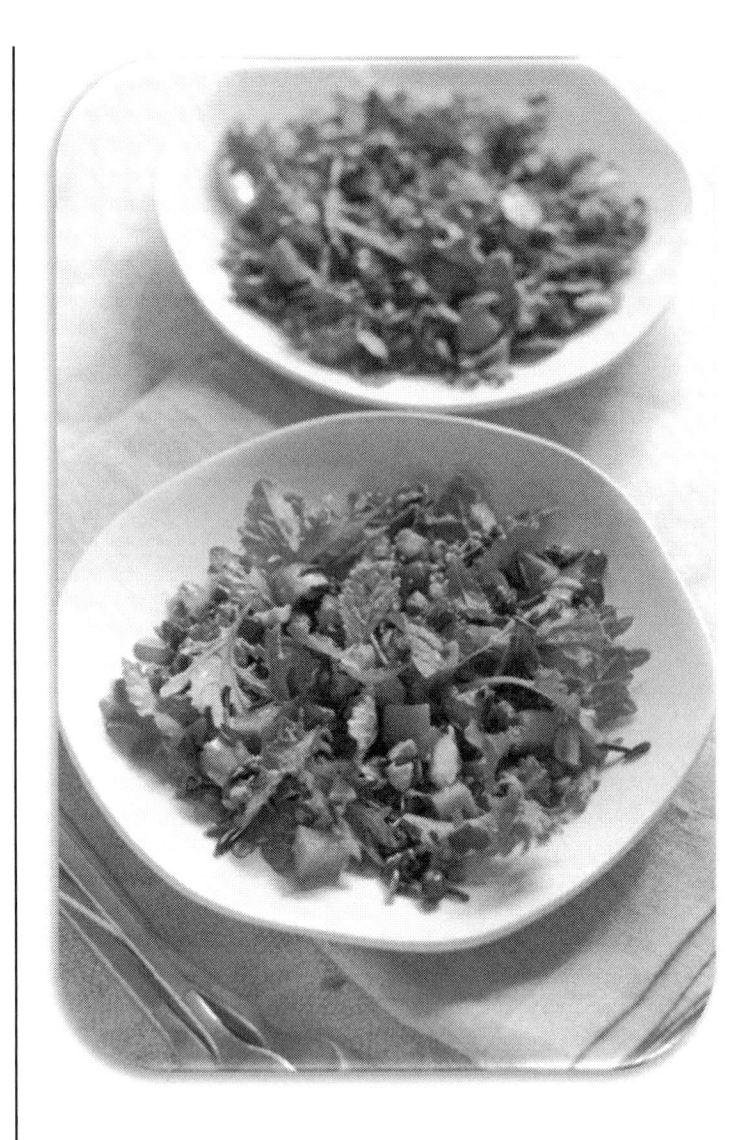

Instructions:

1. Using a blender, combine the honey, olive oil, orange juice, miso paste, and vinegar. Add ground black pepper and salt.
2. Sprinkle the wild rice with the dressing. Add pomegranate seeds, persimmons, and pistachios. Stir thoroughly.

Bulgar Wheat Salad with Chickpea and Pepper

Prep time: 10 minutes

Cooking time: 15 minutes

Servings: 3

Nutrients per serving:

Carbohydrates – 54.9 g

Fat – 23.6 g

Protein – 19.8 g

Calories – 532

Ingredients:

- 4 Tbsp bulgar wheat, cracked
- 4 Tbsp sultanas
- 2 Tbsp red wine vinegar
- 1 tsp caster sugar
- 1 red onion, chopped
- 1 stick celery, diced
- 2 Tbsp olive oil
- 1 red pepper, diced
- 1 cup chickpeas, rinsed and drained
- 1 bunch parsley, chopped
- ¼ cup coriander, chopped
- ½ cup Feta cheese, crumbled

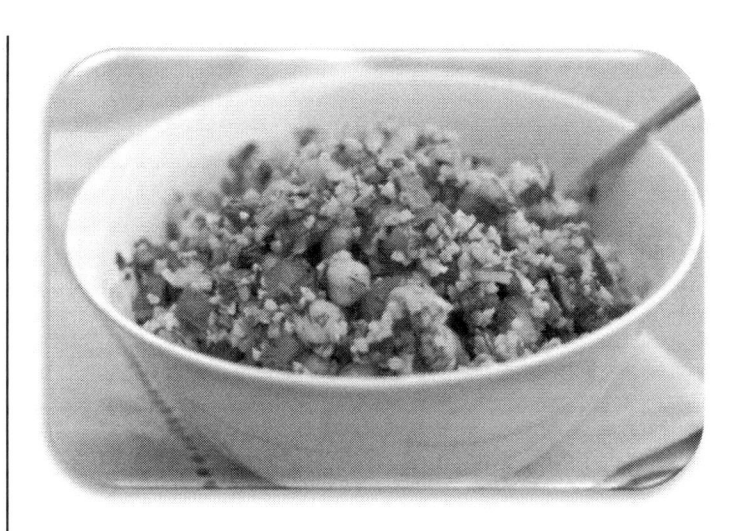

Instructions:

1. Put the bulgar wheat and sultanas in a separate bowl. Pour boiling water over it and leave for 10 minutes.
2. In another bowl, blend the vinegar and sugar. Add the chopped onion, celery, and olive oil. Add salt to taste and stir well.
3. Dry the bulgar and sultanas. Toss the pepper and chickpeas in a bowl and place the bulgar and sultanas into it. Add the onion mixture, feta cheese, and the herbs. Mix thoroughly and serve.

Broad Bean Salad with Barley and Mint

Prep time: 20 minutes

Cooking time: 30 minutes

Servings: 5

Nutrients per serving:

Carbohydrates – 42 g

Fat – 26 g

Protein – 18 g

Calories – 469

Ingredients:

- 1l vegetable stock
- 500g broad beans, podded fresh or frozen
- 225g pearl barley
- 2 handfuls mint leaves
- 200g radish, sliced
- 100g whole hazelnut, roasted and chopped
- 140g goat's cheese, crumbled

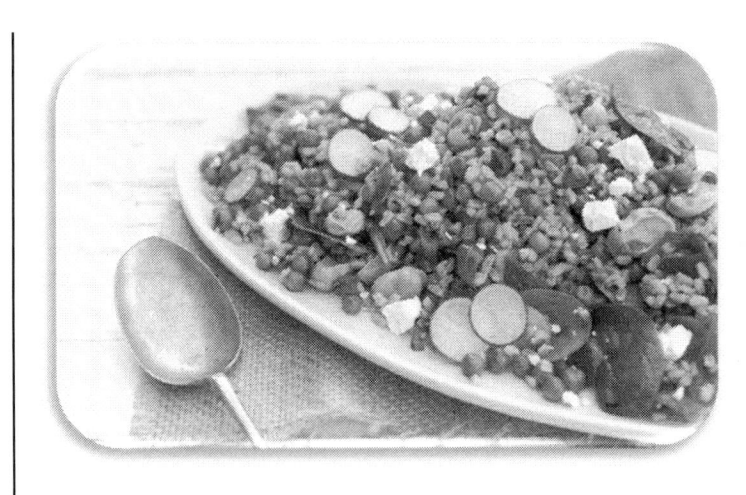

Instructions:

1. Cook the broad beans for 3 minutes. Add the pearl barley to the saucepan and simmer for 40-45 minutes. Dry the barley and mix with chopped mint leaves.
2. Add sliced radish, hazelnut and goat's cheese to the salad. Stir well and serve.

Lentil Salad with Avocado and Feta

Prep time: 5 minutes

Cooking time: 5 minutes

Servings: 2

Nutrients per serving:

Carbohydrates – 31.5 g

Fat – 34.6 g

Protein – 24.4 g

Calories – 558

Ingredients:

- 1 pouch lentil, ready-cooked
- 2 Tbsp red wine vinegar
- 2 Tbsp olive oil
- ½ tsp Dijon mustard
- ½ red onion, chopped
- 2 sticks celery, diced
- ¼ cucumber, diced
- ½ avocado, diced
- ½ cup Feta cheese, crumbled
- 1 handful basil, shredded
- 1 Tbsp flower seeds
- Salt, to taste

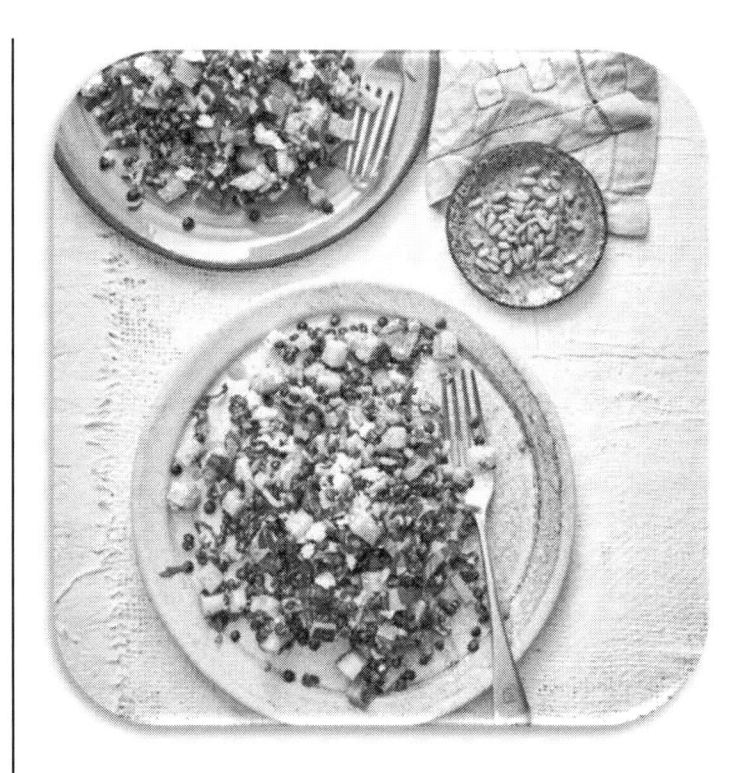

Instructions:

1. Cook the lentils using the packet instructions. Stir the olive oil, vinegar, mustard, and salt in a bowl. Whisk thoroughly and add this mixture to the lentils.
2. Put the diced avocado, cucumber, feta cheese, onion, celery, and basil into the bowl. Blend well and serve with sunflower seeds.

Warm Salad with Cauliflower

Prep time: 15 minutes

Cooking time: 20 minutes

Servings: 4

Nutrients per serving:

Carbohydrates – 19 g

Fat – 11 g

Protein – 8 g

Calories – 206

Ingredients:

- 1 cauliflower, divided into florets
- 2 Tbsp olive oil
- 1 red onion, sliced
- 3 Tbsp sherry vinegar
- 1½ Tbsp honey
- 3 Tbsp raisins
- 3 Tbsp almond, toasted and flaked
- 50g baby spinach

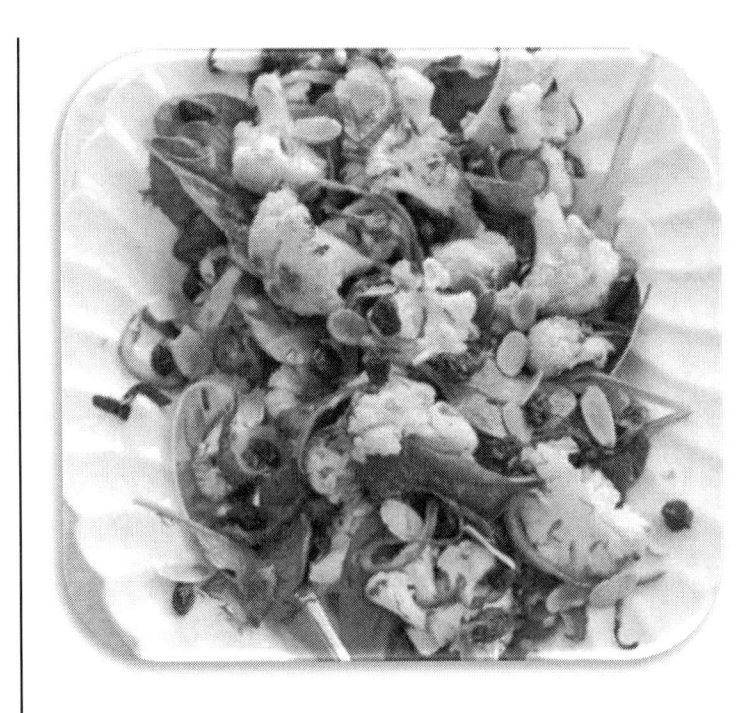

Instructions:

1. Sprinkle the cauliflower with olive oil and toss. Put in the oven already preheated to 180°C. Bake for 15 minutes. Add the red onion to the cauliflower and roast for 15 minutes more.
2. In a separate bowl, combine the vinegar, raisins and honey.
3. Pour the honey mixture over the cooked cauliflower. Add the almonds and spinach and serve.

Soft Tahini Dressing

Prep time: 5 minutes

Cooking time: 0 minutes

Servings: 4

Nutrients per serving:

Carbohydrates – 8.1 g

Fat – 10.8 g

Protein – 3.6 g

Calories – 133

Ingredients:

- ⅓ cup tahini
- 3 Tbsp lemon juice
- 2 Tbsp. maple syrup
- 1 clove garlic, minced
- 6 Tbsp water
- Salt, to taste

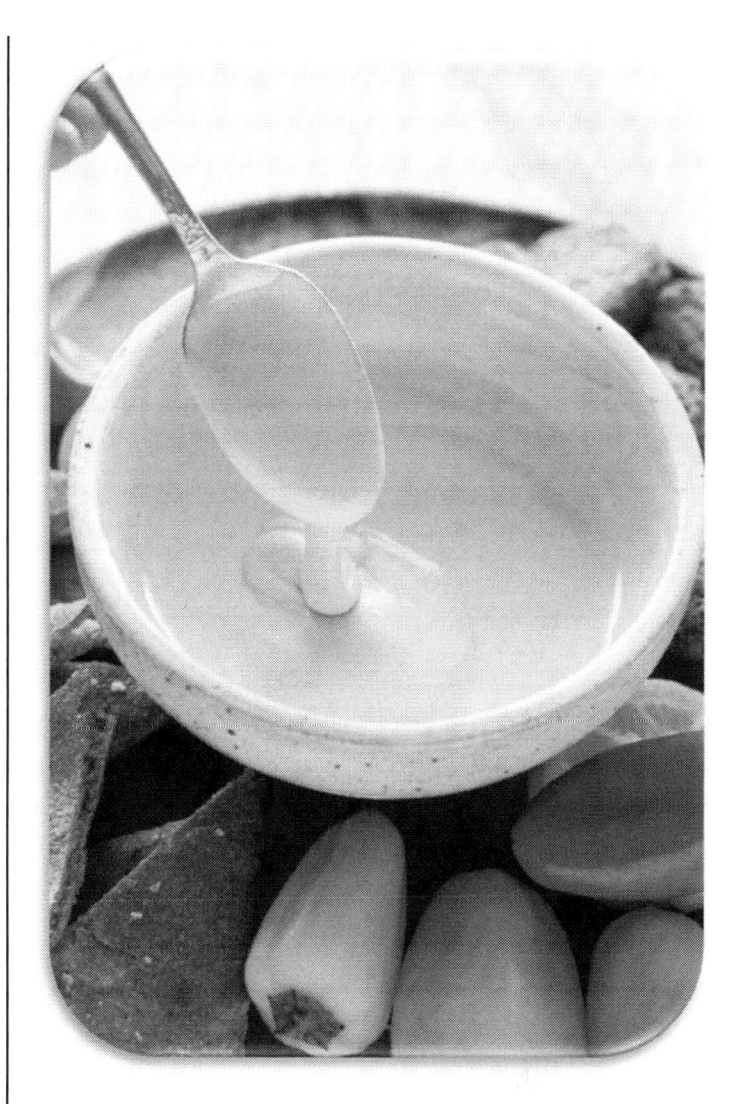

Instructions:

1. Mix the tahini, lemon juice, maple syrup, garlic and salt in a separate bowl. Whisk well.
2. Pour in the water and stir until it is a creamy texture.
3. Serve with your favorite salads.

Lemon Mint Dressing

Prep time: 3 minutes

Cooking time: 0 minutes

Servings: 8

Nutrients per serving:

Carbohydrates – 4.6 g

Fat – 14 g

Protein – 0.1 g

Calories – 138

Ingredients:

- ½ cup lemon juice
- ½ cup extra-virgin olive oil
- ½ cup fresh mint leaves, packed
- 2 Tbsp maple syrup
- ½ Tbsp Dijon mustard
- 1 tsp Himalayan pink salt

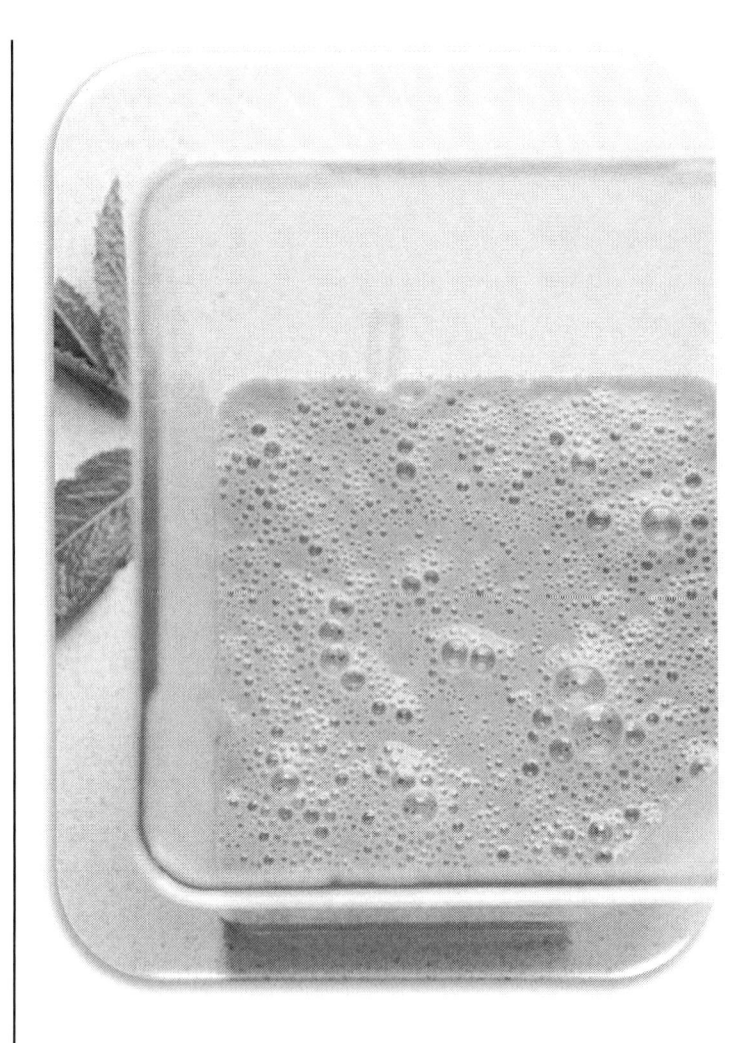

Instructions:

1. Using a blender, mix all the ingredients.
2. Serve with your favorite salads.

SOUPS & STEWS

Chunky Chickpea Soup

Prep time: 15 minutes

Cooking time: 40 minutes

Servings: 3

Nutrients per serving:

Carbohydrates – 26 g

Fat – 2 g

Protein – 4 g

Calories – 142

Ingredients:

- 1 Tbsp olive oil
- 2 leeks, sliced
- 1 clove fresh garlic, minced
- 1½ carrot, sliced
- 1½ stalks celery, chopped
- 1½ cups potatoes, chopped
- ¼ tsp black pepper
- 4 cups vegetable broth
- ½ sprig fresh rosemary
- 1½ sprigs fresh thyme
- 1 bay leaf
- 1 cup fresh kale, chopped
- 1 can chickpea
- Salt, to taste

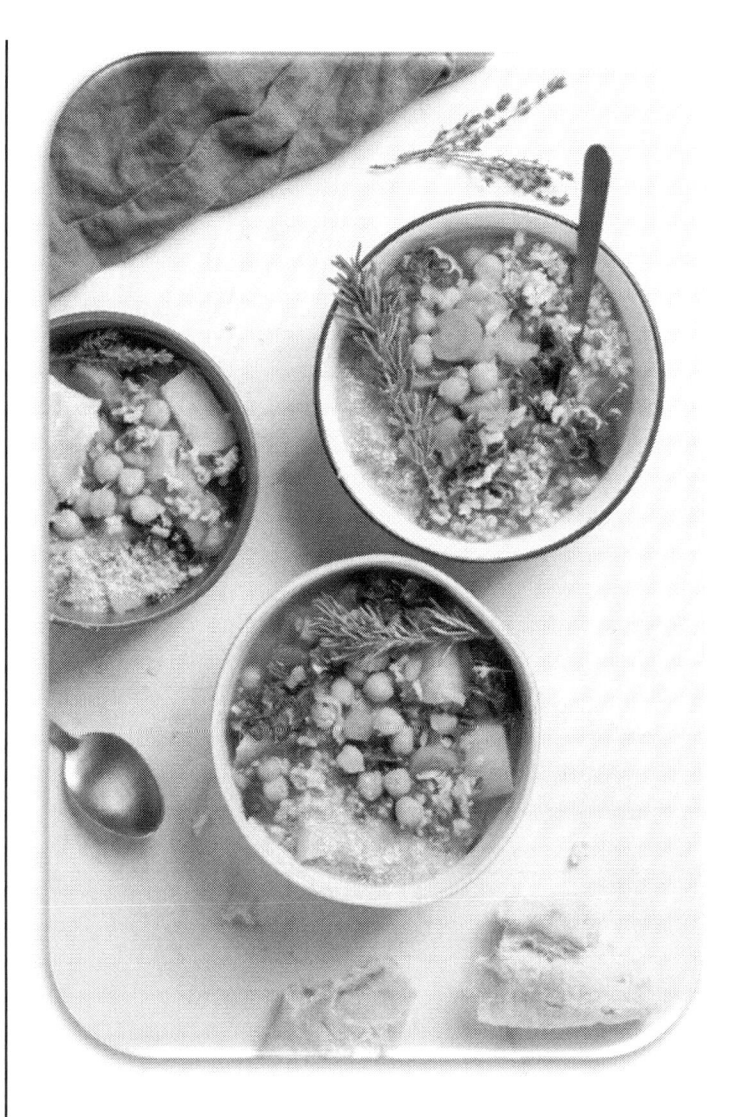

Instructions:

1. Boil the leeks and garlic in a pot until they are soft and fragrant.
2. Put the chopped carrot, celery, potatoes, and black pepper into the pot. Stir well and continue boiling for about 5 minutes.
3. Add the vegetable broth, rosemary, thyme, and bay leaf. Simmer for 20 minutes more.
4. Add kale and chickpeas to the pot and cook for 5 minutes.
5. Take out the rosemary, thyme, bay leaf and serve.

Moroccan Carrot Soup with Cilantro

Prep time: 15 minutes

Cooking time: 10 minutes

Servings: 6

Nutrients per serving:

Carbohydrates – 22.6 g

Fat – 8.2 g

Protein – 5.8 g

Calories –239

Ingredients:

- 5 cups vegetable broth
- 3 cups carrot, cooked and diced
- 1 tsp salt
- 1 tsp ground cumin
- ½ tsp ground coriander
- ½ tsp ground cinnamon
- ¼ tsp ground allspice
- ¼ cup cilantro, chopped
- ¼ tsp cayenne pepper
- 1 cup plain low-fat yoghurt
- ½ cup pepitas, toasted
- 6 Tbsp olive oil
- Freshly ground pepper, to taste

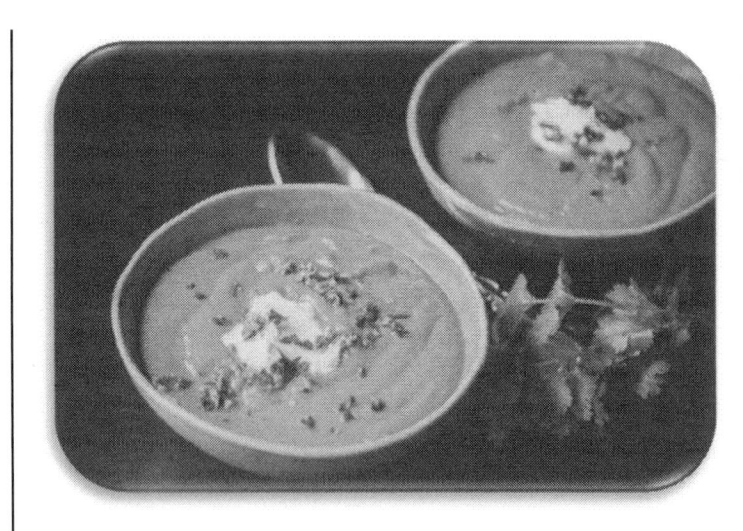

Instructions:

1. Using a food processor, combine the carrots and vegetable broth until smooth.
2. Pour the carrot mixture into a pot, add salt and spices. Sauté for 8-10 minutes. Add ½ cup of water if needed.
3. Drizzle the soup mixture with olive oil and ground pepper.
4. Top your soup with yoghurt, pepitas and chopped cilantro.

Cold Cucumber Soup with Dill

Prep time: 15 minutes

Cooking time: 20 minutes

Servings: 6

Nutrients per serving:

Carbohydrates – 12 g

Fat – 5 g

Protein – 0 g

Calories – 135

Ingredients:

- 2 cups Greek yoghurt
- 1 cup vegetable broth
- 2 cucumbers, diced
- 4 green onions, chopped
- 12 sprigs fresh dill
- 3 Tbsp fresh parsley, chopped
- 4 Tbsp lemon juice
- 2 tsp salt

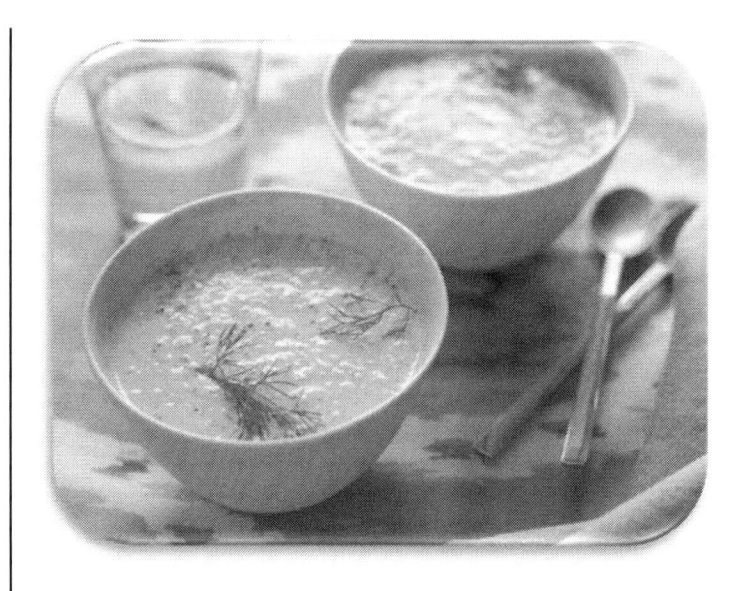

Instructions:

1. In a separate bowl, combine the yoghurt and vegetable broth. Put it aside.
2. Use a food processor to mix the diced cucumbers, chopped parsley and green onions.
3. Blend the cucumber mixture and yoghurt mixture. Add lemon juice and stir well.
4. Place in the fridge for 20 minutes.
5. Serve each portion with 2 sprigs of dill.

Fresh Tomato Avocado Soup with Basil

Prep time: 3 minutes

Cooking time: 0 minutes

Servings: 4

Nutrients per serving:

Carbohydrates – 19 g

Fat – 37 g

Protein – 16 g

Calories – 400

Ingredients:

- 7 large tomatoes, halved, seeded and chopped
- ¼ cup red onion, chopped
- ¼ cup seedless cucumber, chopped
- ¼ cup red bell pepper, sliced
- 1 clove garlic
- 2 Tbsp extra-virgin olive oil
- 1 Tbsp red wine vinegar
- 1 Tbsp salt
- ½ tsp cumin
- ½ tsp cayenne pepper
- 2 avocados, sliced
- ½ cup basil, chopped

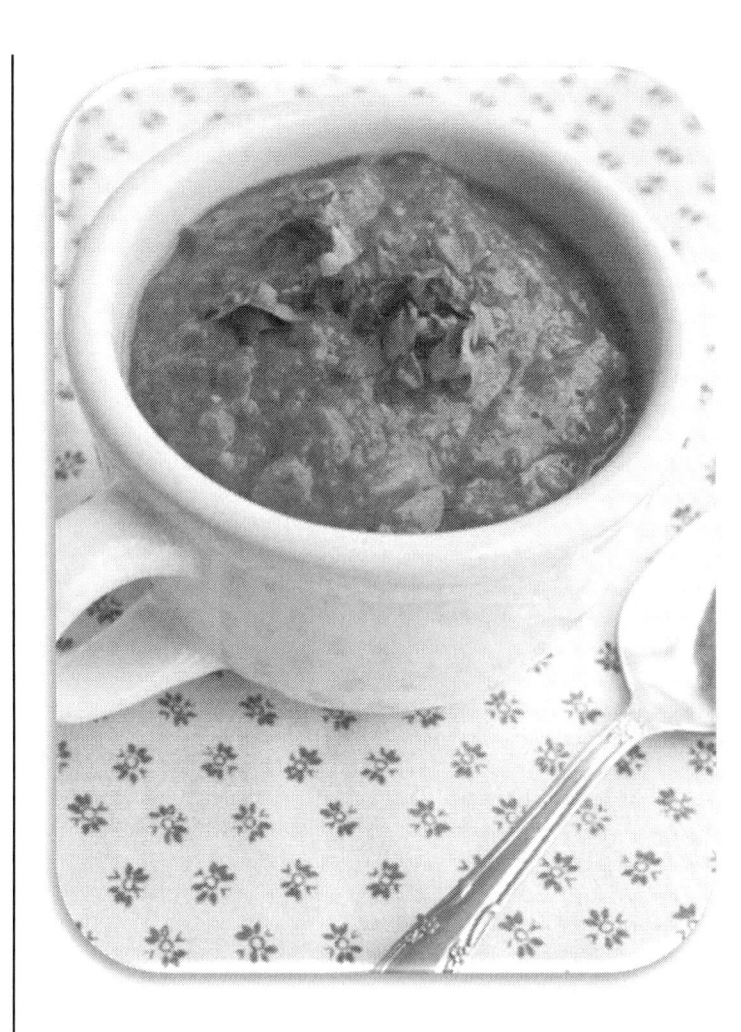

Instructions:

1. Use a food processor to mix all the ingredients you have. Add 1 cup of water and place into the fridge for 1 hour.
2. Top with chopped basil and serve.

Hearty Potato Stew

Prep time: 20 minutes

Cooking time: 30 minutes

Servings: 10

Nutrients per serving:

Carbohydrates – 58.6 g

Fat – 24.1 g

Protein – 7.7 g

Calories – 470

Ingredients:

- 8 large potatoes, peeled and sliced
- 4 large carrots, diced
- 3 quarts water
- 2 stalks celery, chopped
- 2 small onions, chopped
- ¼ cup butter
- 2 Tbsp all-purpose flour
- 1½ tsp salt
- 1 tsp ground black pepper
- 2 cups heavy cream

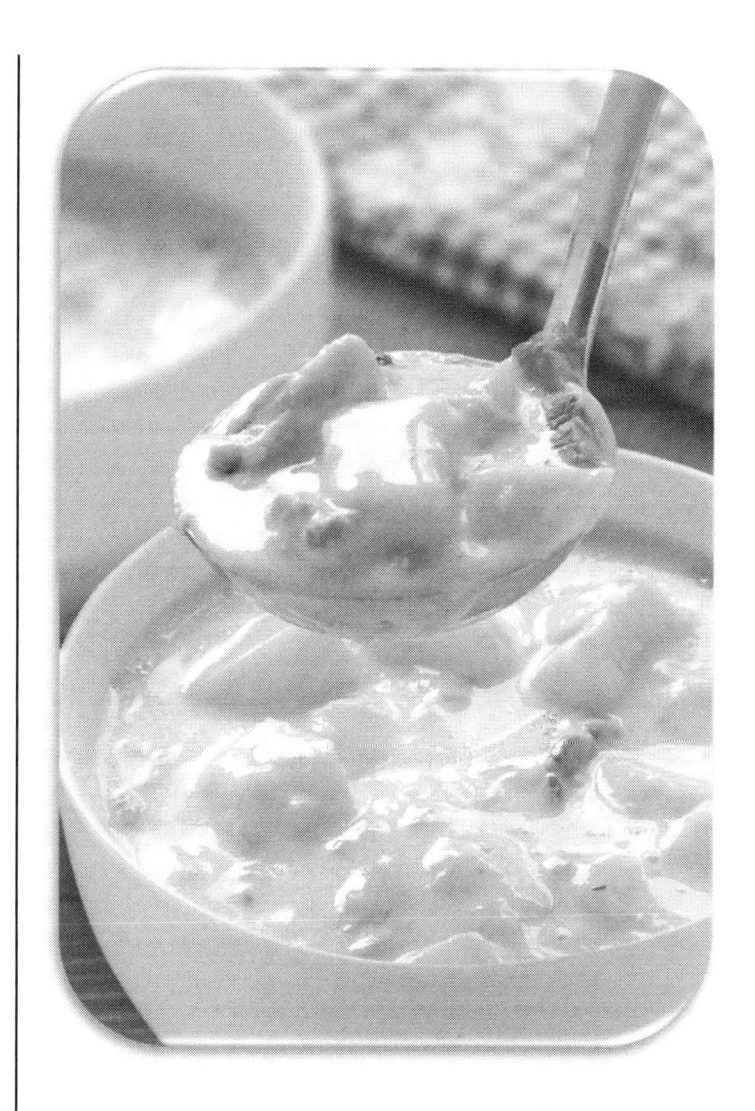

Instructions:

1. Put the potatoes, carrots, and celery in a saucepan with boiling water. Cook for 15 minutes. Drain and put aside. Don't forget to keep the liquid.
2. Place the butter in a pot and cook the onions for 10 minutes until they are tender. Add the flour, heavy cream, salt, and pepper. Stir in the potato mixture and reserved cooking water. Simmer for about 5 minutes and serve.

Indian Stew with Peanuts

Prep time: 15 minutes

Cooking time: 30 minutes

Servings: 6

Nutrients per serving:

Carbohydrates – 54.6 g

Fat – 26.2 g

Protein – 16.1 g

Calories – 504

Ingredients:

- 2 cups rice, uncooked
- 6 cups water
- 1 Tbsp olive oil
- 1 large white onion, chopped
- 4 cloves garlic, minced
- 3 Tbsp fresh ginger root, grated
- 1 can tomatoes with juice, diced
- 1 cup peanuts, toasted and sliced
- 1 eggplant, peeled and cut into cubes
- ½ lemon, sliced
- 1 handful coriander
- Salt and pepper, to taste

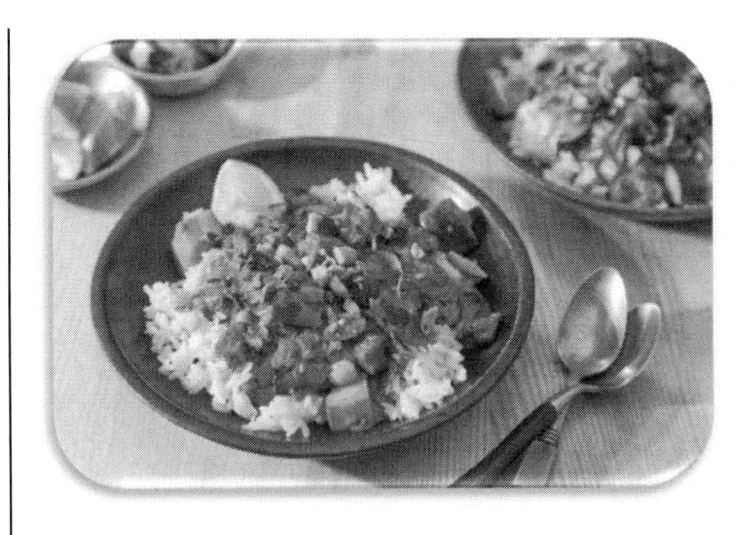

Instructions:

1. Boil the rice for about 20 minutes.
2. Fry the onion in the pan. Add the grated ginger and minced garlic to the pan and fry for 5 minutes more. Mix in the tomatoes, eggplant cubes, peanuts, salt and pepper. Simmer for 5 minutes.
3. Cover the rice with the tomato mixture. Top with coriander leaves and a lemon slice.

MAIN COURSES

Cream Cheese Leek Risotto

Prep time: 5 minutes

Cooking time: 30 minutes

Servings: 3

Nutrients per serving:

Carbohydrates – 74 g

Fat – 63 g

Protein – 17 g

Calories –977

Ingredients:

- 1 cup risotto rice, rinsed
- 3-4 cups vegetable broth
- 1 leek, chopped
- 1 onion, diced
- 3 Tbsp olive oil
- 1 cup peas, frozen
- ¾ cup cream
- ¾ cup cream cheese
- 3 Tbsp soy sauce
- ½ tsp salt
- ½ tsp pepper

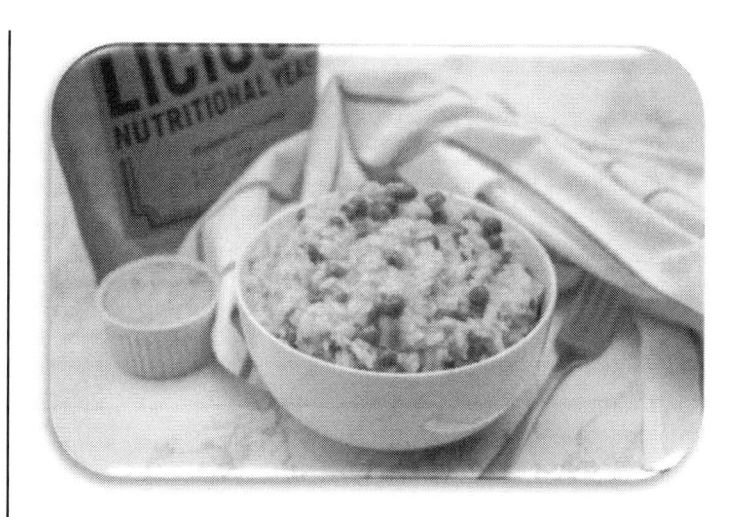

Instructions:

1. Fry the leek and onion in the pan in olive oil for 5 minutes. Add the risotto rice and cook for 2 more minutes.
2. Pour ¾ vegetable broth into the pan and cook for 20 minutes.
3. Mix in the frozen peas, cream, cream cheese, and soy sauce. Stir thoroughly and cook for 5 minutes.
4. Add salt and pepper to taste and serve.

Broccoli Pesto Fusilli

Prep time: 10minutes

Cooking time: 5 minutes

Servings: 4

Nutrients per serving:

Carbohydrates – 79 g

Fat – 26 g

Protein – 19 g

Calories – 427

Ingredients:

- 12 oz fusilli pasta
- 12 oz broccoli florets, frozen
- 2 cloves garlic, minced
- ½ cup fresh basil leaves, chopped
- 3 Tbsp olive oil
- ½ cup water
- 1 Tbsp lemon zest, grated
- ½ cup almonds, toasted and sliced
- ¼ cup parmesan cheese, grated
- Kosher salt, to taste

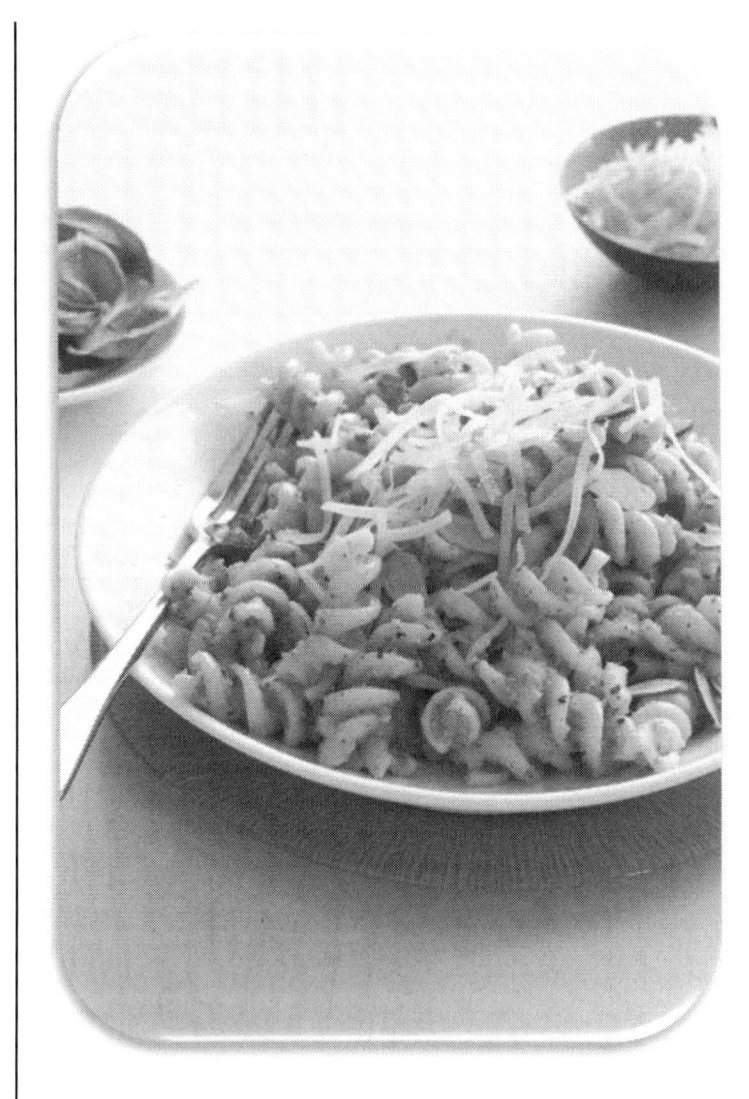

Instructions:

1. Cook the fusilli pasta according to the package instructions. Reserve ½ cup of pasta cooking water. Drain the fusilli pasta and put it aside.
2. Mix the broccoli, minced garlic, and ½ cup of water in a bowl. Heat in the microwave for 5 minutes. Add basil, salt, oil and lemon zest. Using a food processor blend this mixture until smooth.
3. Combine the pasta with the pesto and pour in the ½ cup of reserved cooking liquid. Top with almonds and parmesan.

Noodles with Carrot and Sesame

Prep time: 10 minutes

Cooking time: 10minutes

Servings: 2

Nutrients per serving:

Carbohydrates – 105 g

Fat – 6.5 g

Protein – 26 g

Calories –545

Ingredients:

- 9 oz noodles
- 1 carrot, grated
- 1 thumb ginger, fresh and diced
- 3 spring onions, chopped
- 1 chili, diced
- 2 Tbsp spicy sauce
- 2 Tbsp soy sauce
- 2 eggs
- 1 clove garlic, minced
- 4 Tbsp sesame seeds
- Salt, to taste

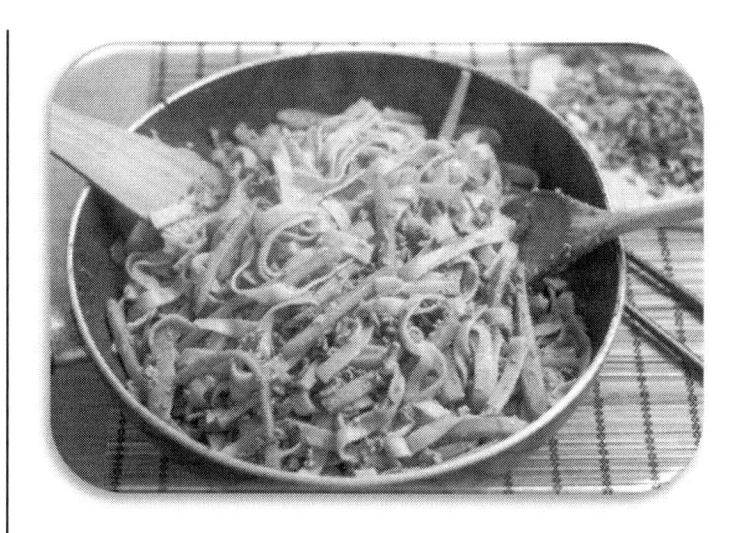

Instructions:

1. Boil noodles according to the package instruction.
2. Put the carrots, ginger, garlic, spring onions, and chili in the pan. Fry for 3-4 minutes. Gently stir when frying.
3. Beat the eggs and stir them.
4. Pour the egg mixture into the pan. Mix thoroughly and cook for 2 more minutes.
5. Add salt and sauces.
6. Top the noodles with sesame seeds and serve.

Linguine with Mushrooms

Prep time: 10 minutes

Cooking time: 10 minutes

Servings: 6

Nutrients per serving:

Carbohydrates – 62 g

Fat – 15 g

Protein – 15 g

Calories – 430

Ingredients:

- 1 lb linguine
- 6 Tbsp olive oil
- 12 oz mixed mushrooms, sliced
- 3 cloves garlic, chopped
- ¼ cup nutritional yeast
- 2 green onions, sliced
- Salt and ground pepper, to taste

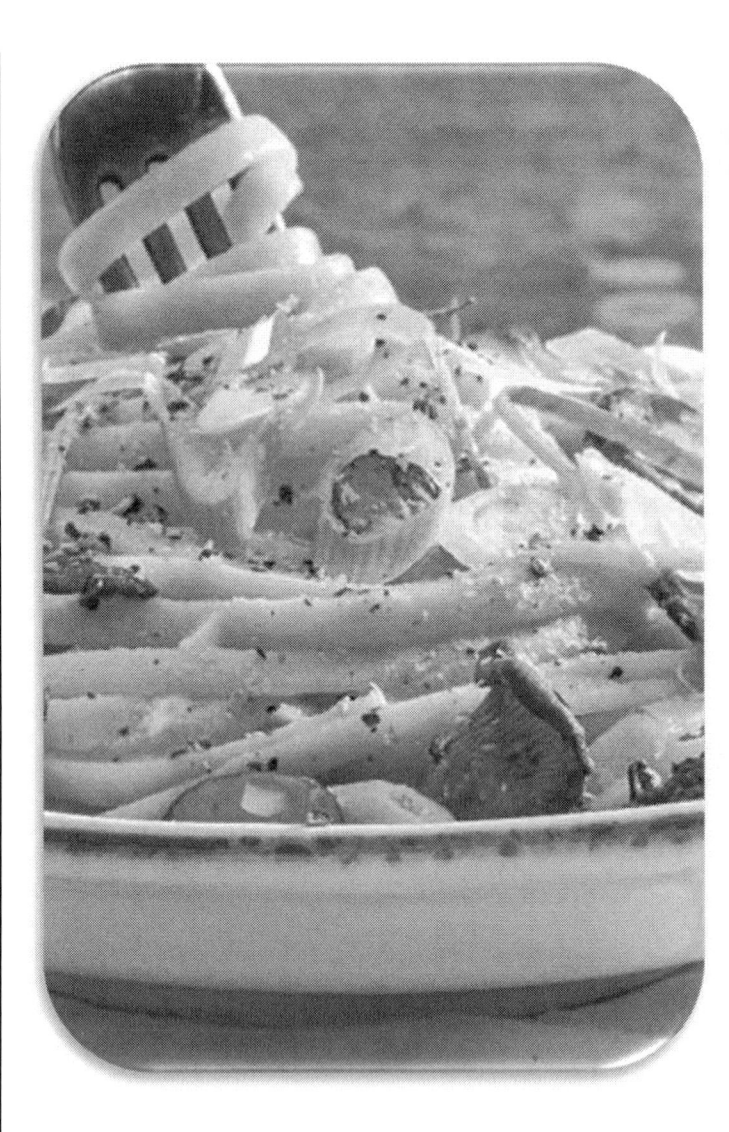

Instructions:

1. Cook linguine according to the package instructions. Reserve ¾ of the linguine cooking water. Drain the linguine and put it aside.
2. Add sliced mushrooms and garlic to the pan and fry for 5 minutes until they are browned.
3. Put the mushrooms on the linguine. Add the nutritional yeast, reserved water, salt, and pepper. Stir well and serve.

Marinated Tofu with Peanuts

Prep time: 20minutes

Cooking time: 30 minutes

Servings: 4

Nutrients per serving:

Carbohydrates – 12 g

Fat – 25 g

Protein – 32 g

Calories –400

Ingredients:

- 2 14-ounces packages firm tofu, drained and sliced
- 1 jalapeño, with seeds, sliced
- ½ cup soy sauce
- 2 Tbsp light brown sugar
- 2 tsp ginger, peeled and grated
- 2 tsp vegetable oil
- 2 cups bean sprouts, divided
- Kosher salt
- 6 scallions, sliced
- ½ cup peanuts, salted, roasted and chopped
- ¼ cup mint leaves

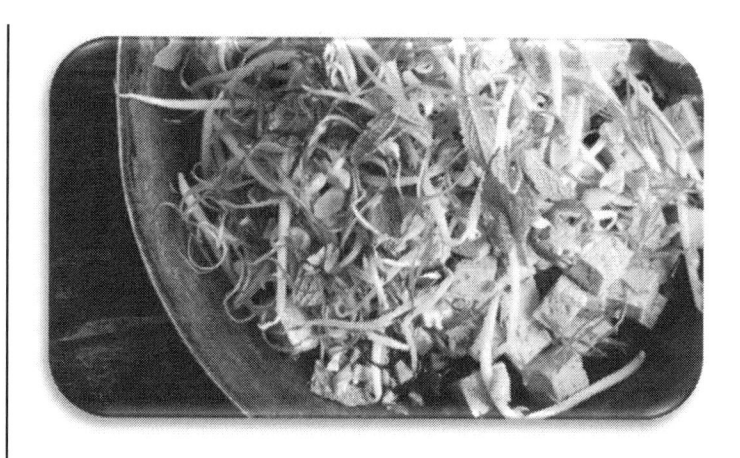

Instructions:

1. In a separate bowl, mix the jalapeño, soy sauce, brown sugar and ginger. Pour this mixture over the tofu and put aside for 30 minutes.
2. Fry the bean sprouts in a pan for 3 minutes. Add salt and all the remaining ingredients, including the marinated tofu.
3. Serve with mint leaves.

DESSERT & FRUIT-FOCUSED MEALS

Sushi with Peanut Butter and Jelly

Prep time: 10 minutes

Cooking time: 0 minutes

Servings: 1

Nutrients per serving:

Carbohydrates – 45 g

Fat – 17 g

Protein – 10 g

Calories – 350

Ingredients:

- 2 Tbsp smooth peanut butter
- 2 slices bread
- 2 Tbsp jelly

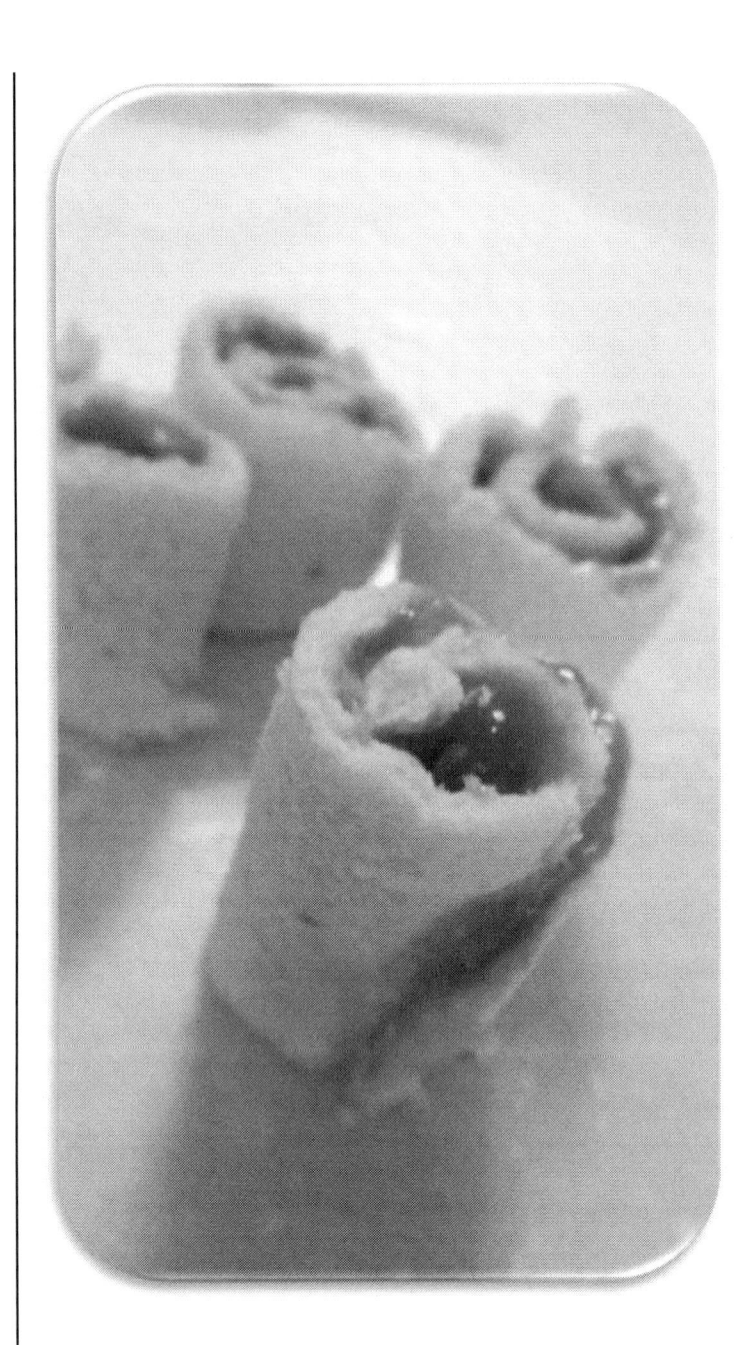

Instructions:

1. Cut the crust from the bread.
2. Squish the bread with the help of a large soup can.
3. Spread 1 Tbsp jelly and 1 Tbsp peanut butter on each bread slice.
4. Roll the slice and divide into 4 pieces.

Apple Dutch Pancake

Prep time: 5 minutes

Cooking time: 20 minutes

Servings: 2

Nutrients per serving:

Carbohydrates – 78.5 g

Fat – 12.7 g

Protein – 14 g

Calories – 447

Ingredients:

- 1 apple, cut into thin slices
- 2 eggs
- 2 Tbsp maple syrup
- 1 Tbsp butter
- ½ cup milk
- 1 tsp cinnamon
- ¼ tsp salt
- 1 tsp lemon zest
- 1 Tbsp lemon juice
- 1 cup whole wheat flour
- ¼ tsp ginger powder (optional)

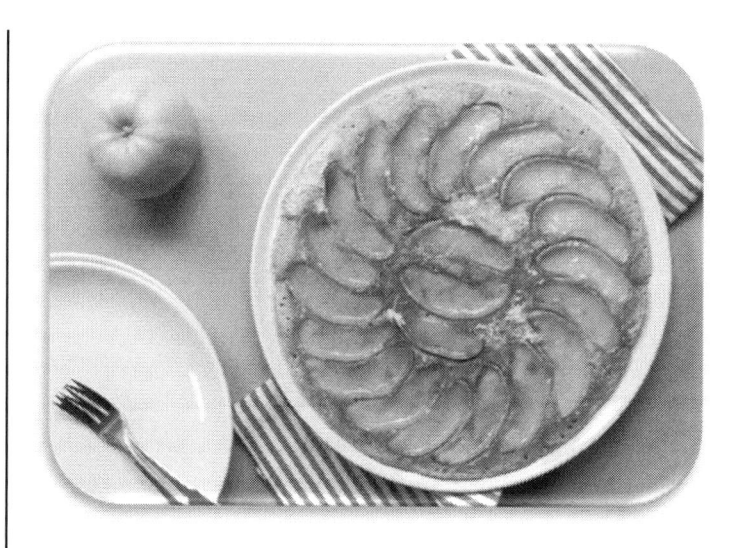

Instructions:

1. Heat the butter in a pan. Add ½ Tbsp maple syrup and put the apple slices in the pan. Caramelize them for about 5 minutes.
2. Make the dough from flour, eggs, milk, cinnamon, salt, lemon juice, lemon zest, and the remaining maple syrup. Add the ginger powder if you want.
3. Put your dough in the pan and cook for about 2 minutes. Then put in the oven (preheated to 180°C) and bake for 12 minutes.

Delicate Banana Pancakes

Prep time: 5 minutes

Cooking time: 10 minutes

Servings: 4

Nutrients per serving:

Carbohydrates – 31 g

Fat – 12 g

Protein – 10 g

Calories – 254

Ingredients:

- 2 ripe bananas
- 2 eggs
- 1 Tbsp almond butter
- 1 tsp baking powder
- 2 Tbsp almond meal
- 2 Tbsp water
- 1 Tbsp nut butter
- Fresh berries (your favorite ones)

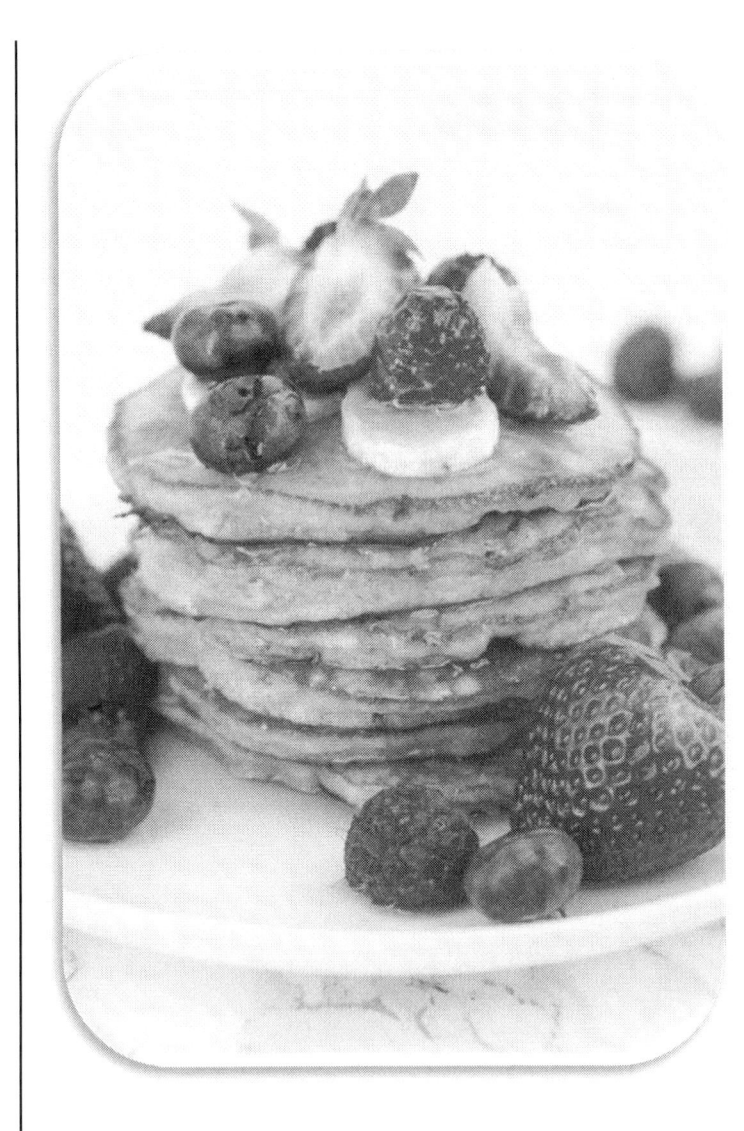

Instructions:

1. Use an electric mixer to blend the bananas and eggs. Add the almond butter, baking powder, almond meal, and water to this mixture and create a creamy batter.
2. Put the batter in the pan (about ¼ cup for each pancake) and cook for 3-4 minutes on each side.
3. Serve with the berries and nut butter.

Baked Banana with Almond Butter

Prep time: 5 minutes

Cooking time: 15 minutes

Servings: 1

Nutrients per serving:

Carbohydrates – 31 g

Fat – 9.4 g

Protein – 4.7 g

Calories – 206

Ingredients:

- 1 banana
- 1 Tbsp almond butter
- ½ tsp cinnamon

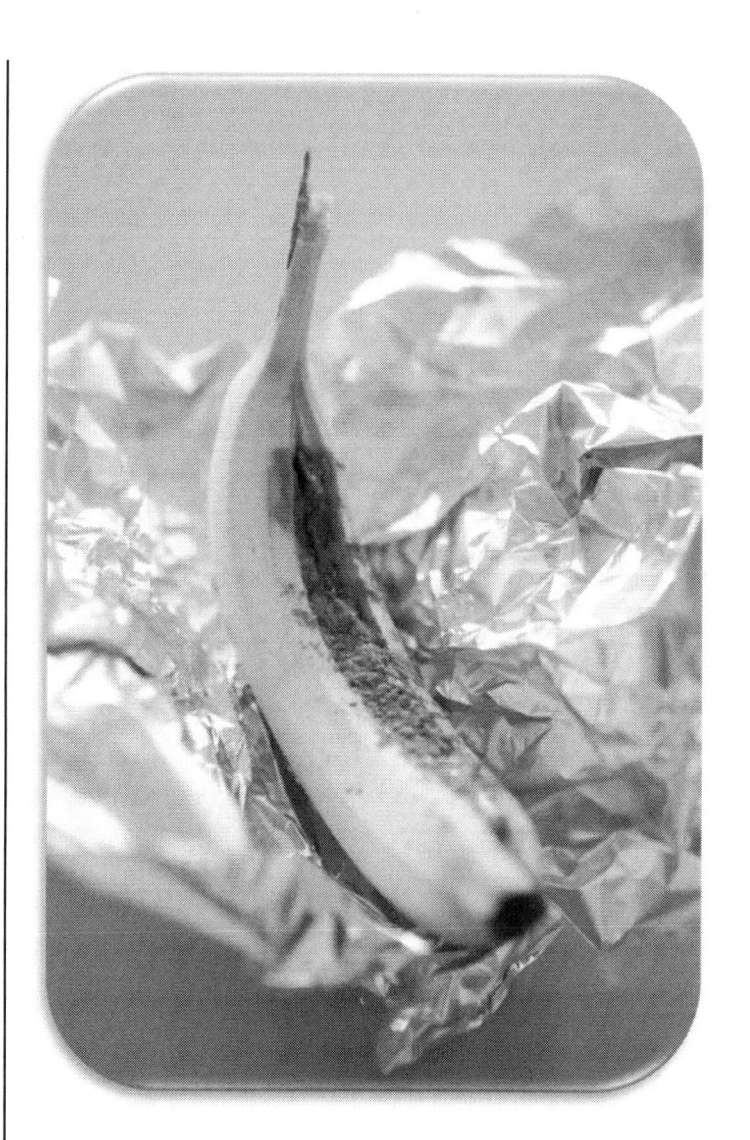

Instructions:

1. Don't peel the banana but slice it lengthwise.
2. Stuff the banana with almond butter and powder with cinnamon.
3. Use aluminum foil to wrap the banana and put it in the oven (preheated to 190°C). Bake for 15 minutes.

Strawberry Cheesecake Toasts

Prep time: 5 minutes

Cooking time: 8 minutes

Servings: 2

Nutrients per serving:

Carbohydrates – 34.3 g

Fat – 16.5 g

Protein – 12.3 g

Calories – 335

Ingredients:

- 2 thick slices of bread
- ½ cup strawberries chopped
- ¼ cup cream cheese
- 2 tsp sugar
- 1 pinch salt
- 2 eggs
- 2 Tbsp milk
- ½ tsp vanilla extract
- ¼ tsp cinnamon
- Oil or butter for cooking

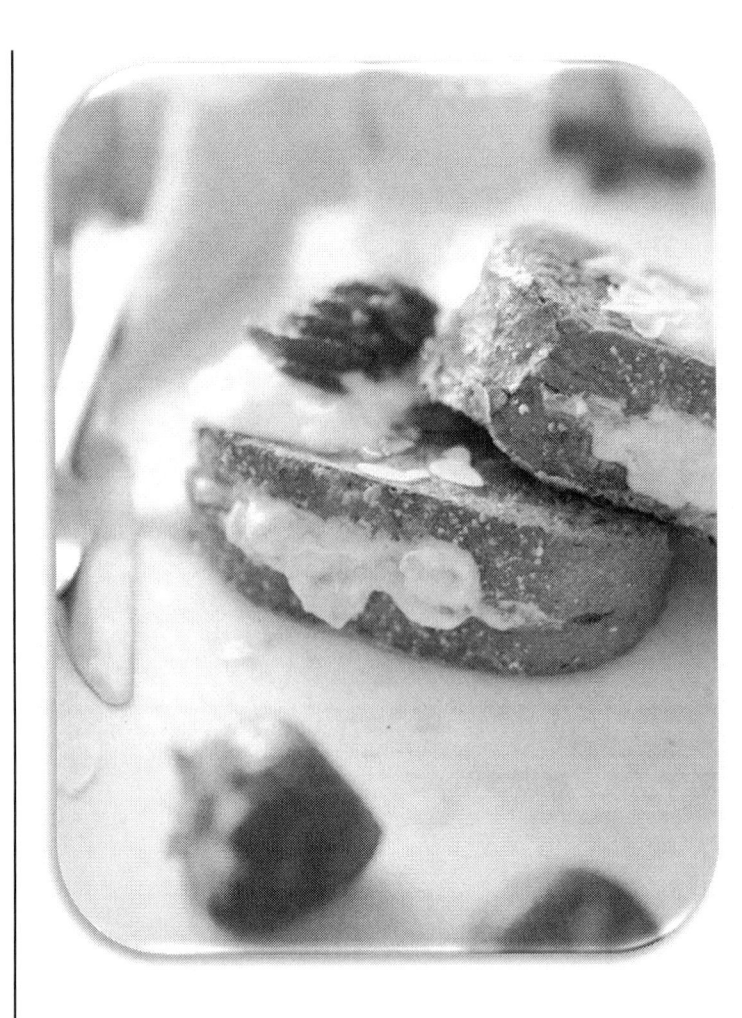

Instructions:

1. Create a pocket in one side of each slice by cutting a slit.
2. Take a bowl and mix the strawberries, cream cheese, sugar and salt. Put the mixture into each bread pocket.
3. Combine the milk, eggs, vanilla and cinnamon. Whisk well.
4. Dunk each stuffed piece into the egg mixture and add it to the frying pan. Fry each side for about 4 minutes.

Raspberry Vanilla Cream

Prep time: 3 minutes

Cooking time: 30 minutes

Servings: 6

Nutrients per serving:

Carbohydrates – 20 g

Fat – 0 g

Protein – 1 g

Calories – 82

Ingredients:

- 3 ripe bananas, frozen and cut into pieces
- 1 cup raspberries, frozen and fresh
- ¼ cup almond milk
- 1 tsp vanilla extract

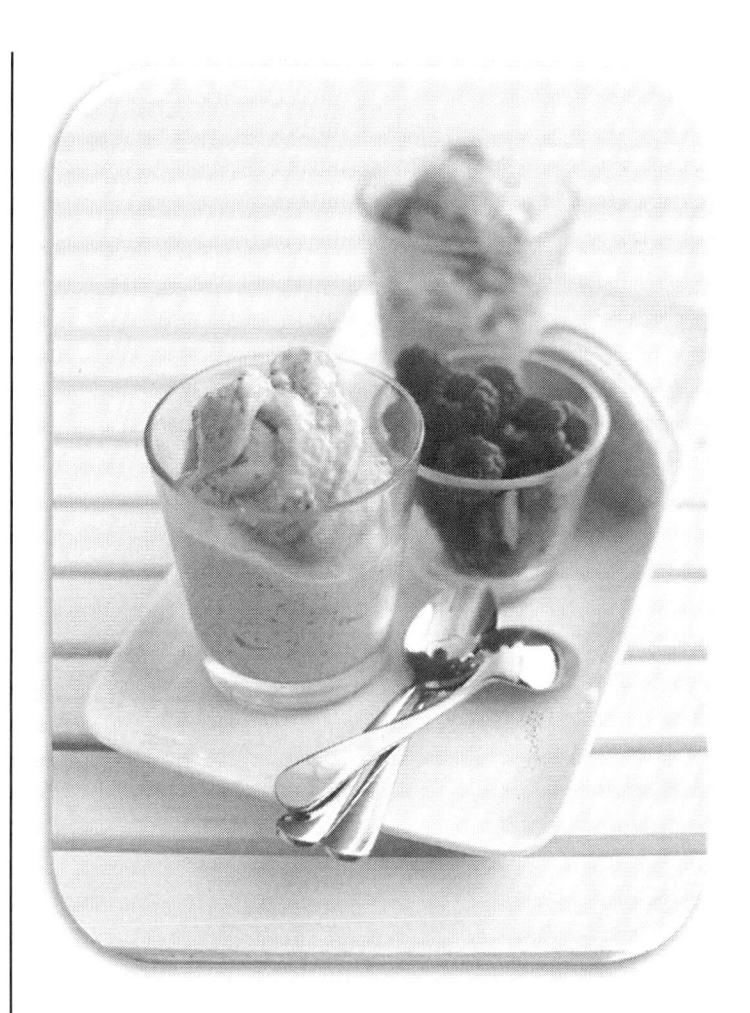

Instructions:

1. Mix all the ingredients in a blender except the fresh raspberries.
2. Cool the mixture in the fridge for 30 minutes.
3. Serve with fresh raspberries.

Coconut Muffins

Prep time: 15 minutes

Cooking time: 30 minutes

Servings: 6

Nutrients per serving:

Carbohydrates – 8 g

Fat – 25 g

Protein – 5 g

Calories – 261

Ingredients:

- 2½ cups coconut milk
- 1¼ cup almond meal
- 2 cups shredded coconut
- 1 tsp salt

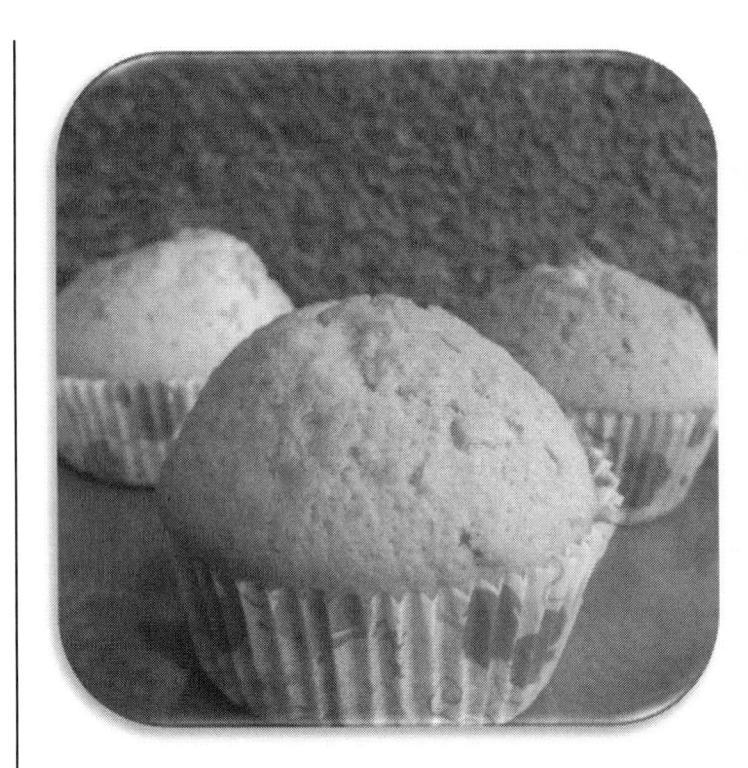

Instructions:

1. Add all the ingredients to a separate bowl and stir until the mixture becomes smooth.
2. Add the batter to the muffin cups and put them in the oven (preheated to 180°C). Cook for about 30 minutes until golden-brown on top.

Splendid Cherry Ice-Cream

Prep time: 15 minutes

Cooking time: 20 minutes

Servings: 8

Nutrients per serving:

Carbohydrates – 18 g

Fat – 7.5 g

Protein – 2.5 g

Calories – 161

Ingredients:

- 4 bananas, cut into pieces and frozen
- 1 cup cherries, frozen
- ½ cup vanilla extract
- 1 Tbsp unsweetened almond milk

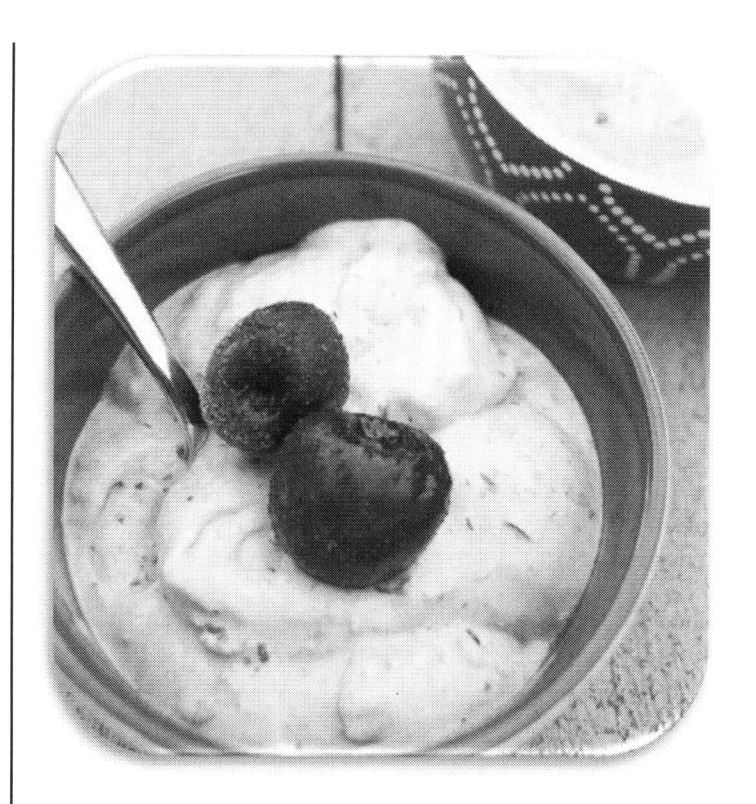

Instructions:

1. Stir the frozen bananas, cherries, and vanilla extract together using a food processor.
2. Add the almond milk and blend until the mixture becomes creamy.
3. Serve your great dessert!

Awesome Chocolate Mousse

Prep time: 10 minutes

Cooking time: 5 minutes

Servings: 3

Nutrients per serving:

Carbohydrates – 8 g

Fat – 24 g

Protein – 8 g

Calories – 259

Ingredients:

- 1 can full-fat coconut milk
- 3 Tbsp raw cocoa powder
- 3 eggs

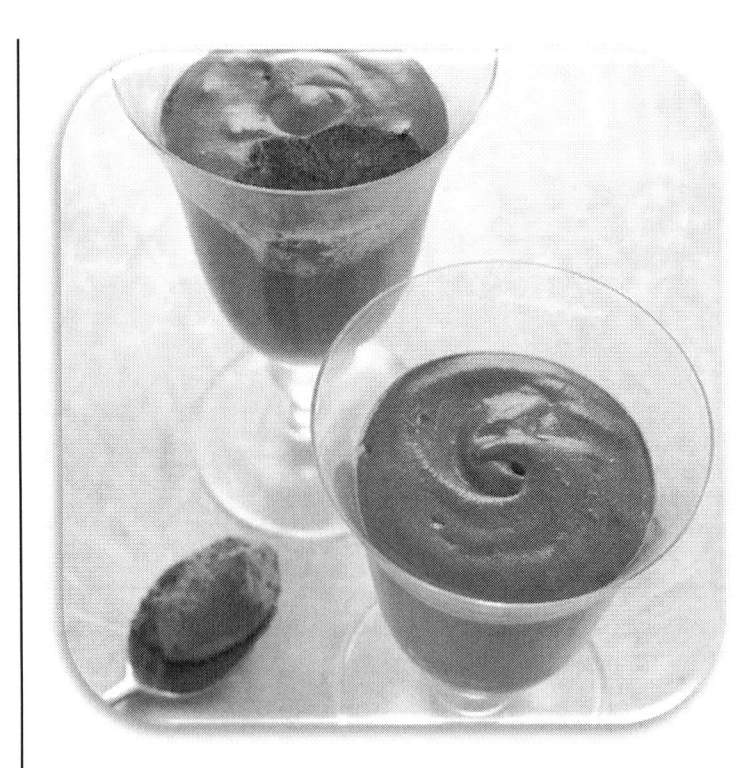

Instructions:

1. Cool the coconut milk in the fridge the night before you want to make this mousse. The next morning, remove only the hardened part of the milk and add this to a stockpot.
2. Add the eggs and cocoa powder and whisk over a low heat until combined and the coconut cream has softened.
3. Chill before serving.

DRINKS & SMOOTHIES

Bracing Coffee Smoothie

Prep time: 5 minutes

Cooking time: 5 minutes

Servings: 1

Nutrients per serving:

Carbohydrates – 46.8 g

Fat – 4.2 g

Protein – 8.1 g

Calories – 245

Ingredients:

- 1 banana, sliced and frozen
- ½ cup strong brewed coffee
- ½ cup milk
- ¼ cup rolled oats
- 1 tsp nut butter

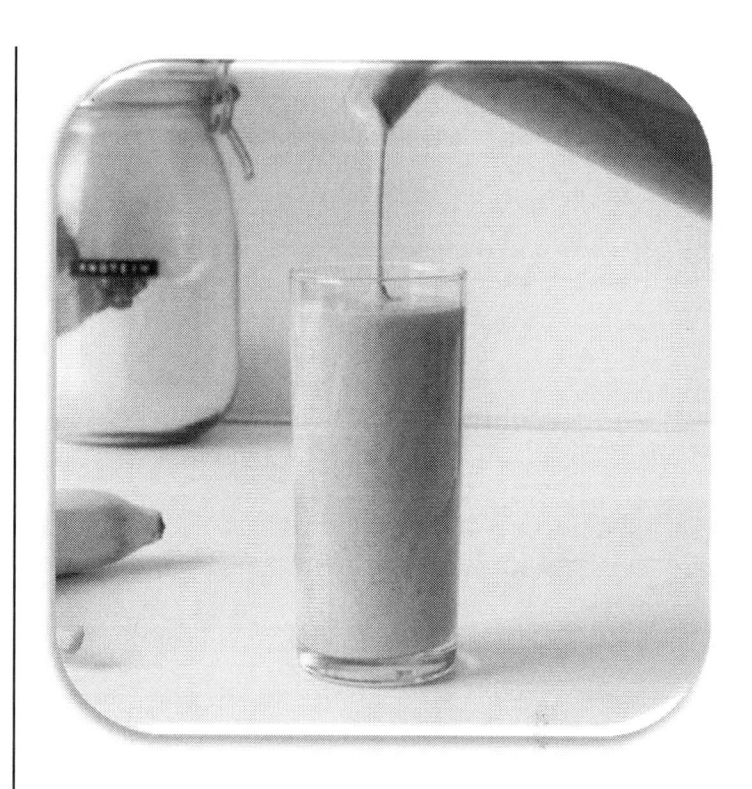

Instructions:

1. Mix all the ingredients until smooth.
2. Enjoy your morning drink!

Vitamin Green Smoothie

Prep time: 5 minutes

Cooking time: 5 minutes

Servings: 2

Nutrients per serving:

Carbohydrates – 41.7 g

Fat – 3.3 g

Protein – 6.2 g

Calories – 202

Ingredients:

- 1 cup milk or juice
- 1 cup spinach or kale
- ½ cup plain yoghurt
- 1 kiwi
- 1 Tbsp chia or flax
- 1 tsp vanilla

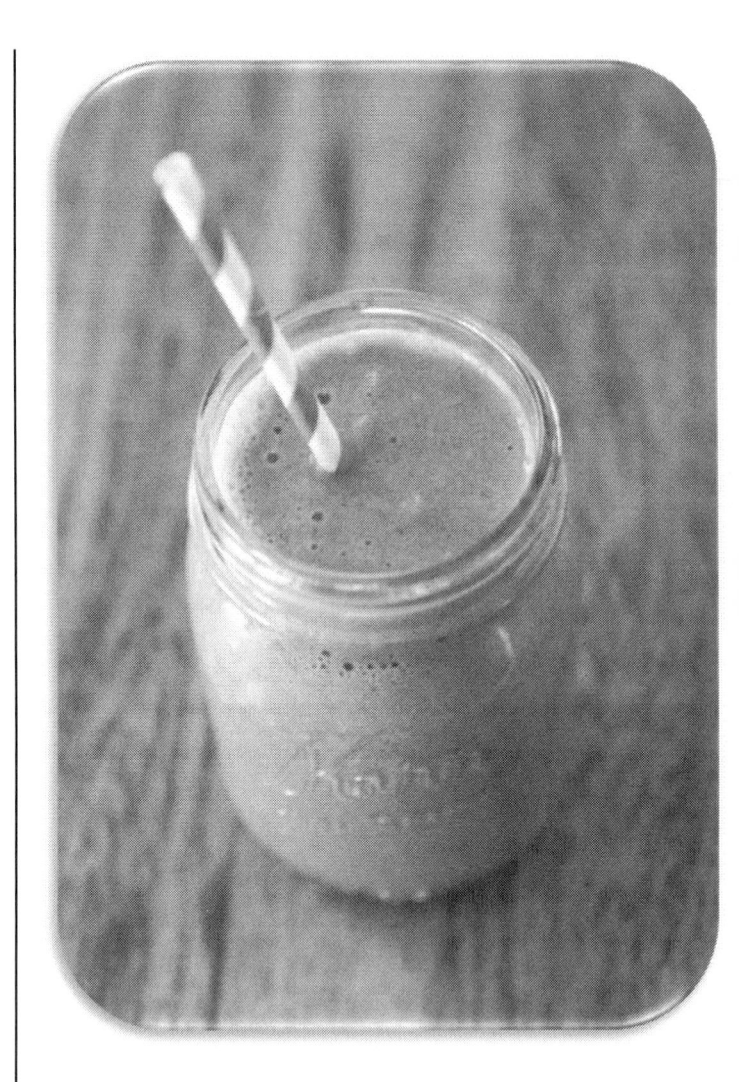

Instructions:

1. Mix the milk or juice and greens until smooth. Add the remaining ingredients and continue blending until smooth again.
2. Enjoy your delicious drink!

Strawberry Grapefruit Smoothie

Prep time: 5 minutes

Cooking time: 5 minutes

Servings: 2

Nutrients per serving:

Carbohydrates – 41.7 g

Fat – 0.7 g

Protein – 2.9 g

Calories – 173

Ingredients:

- 1 banana
- ½ cup strawberries, frozen
- 1 grapefruit
- ¼ cup milk
- ¼ cup plain yoghurt
- 2 Tbsp honey
- ½ tsp ginger, chopped

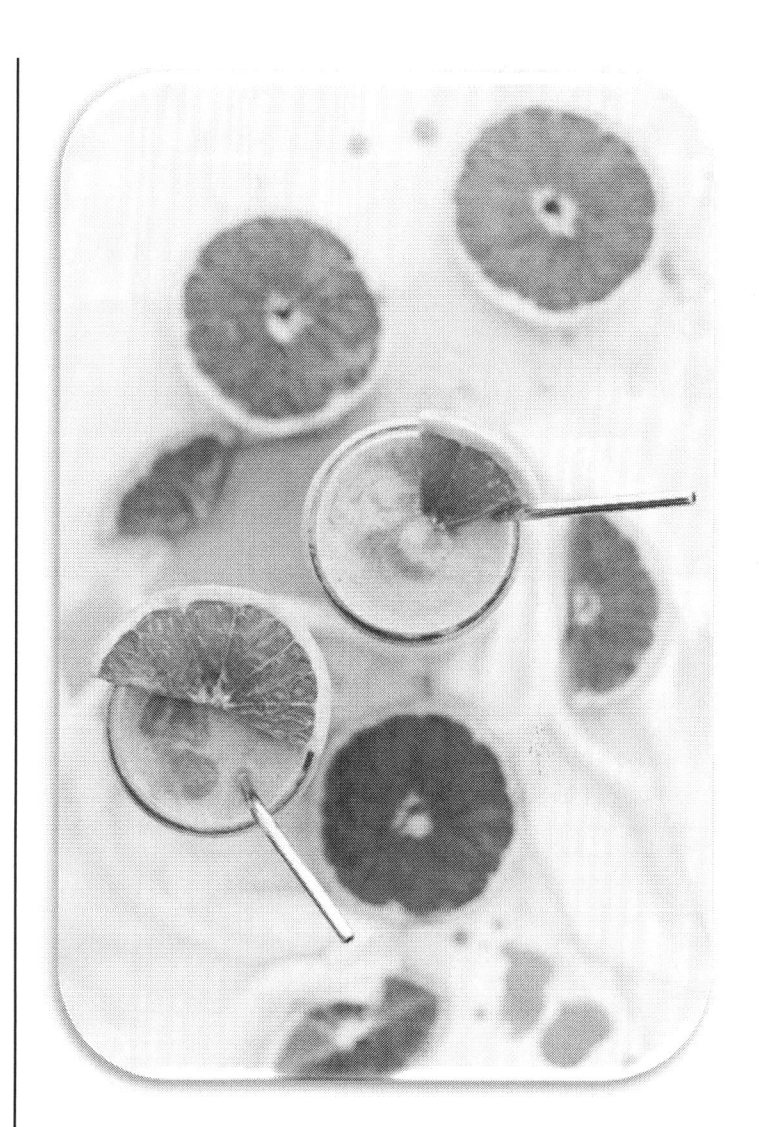

Instructions:

1. Using a mixer, blend all the ingredients.
2. When smooth, top your drink with a slice of grapefruit and enjoy it!

Inspirational Orange Smoothie

Prep time: 5 minutes

Cooking time: 5 minutes

Servings: 1

Nutrients per serving:

Carbohydrates – 60.2 g

Fat – 0.5 g

Protein – 17.2 g

Calories – 297

Ingredients:

- 4 mandarin oranges, peeled
- 1 banana, sliced and frozen
- ½ cup non-fat Greek yoghurt
- ¼ cup coconut water
- 1 tsp vanilla extract
- 5 ice cubes

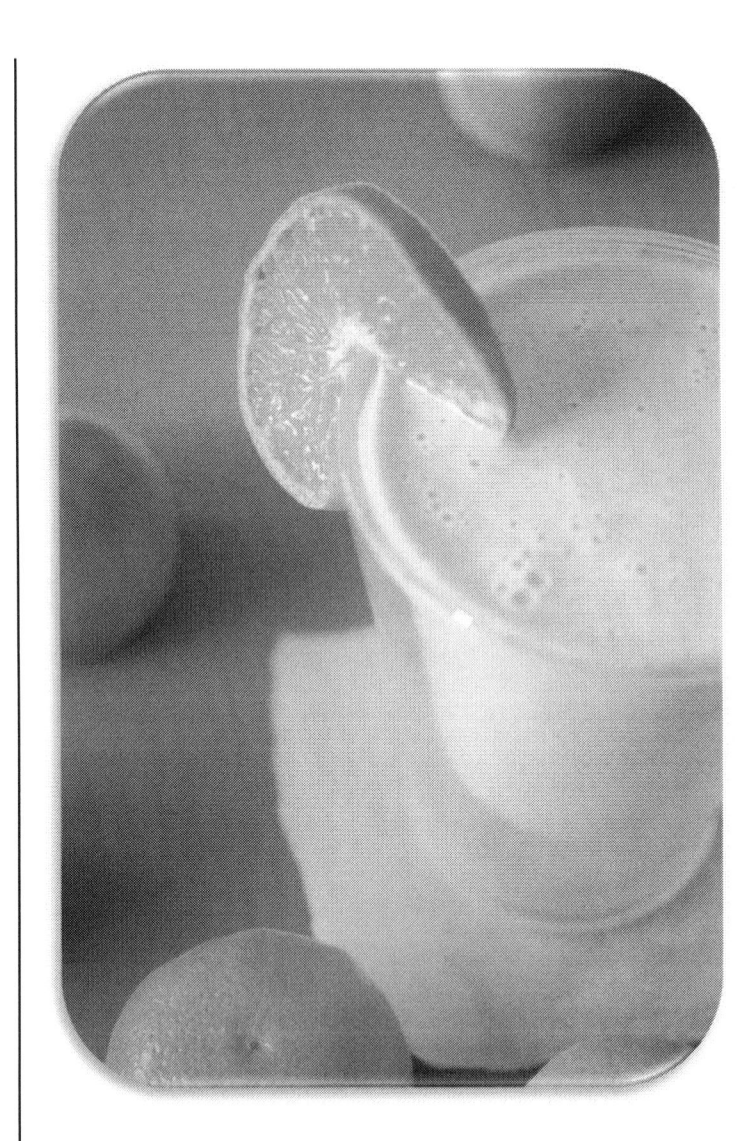

Instructions:

1. Using a mixer, whisk all the ingredients.
2. Enjoy your drink!

Simple Avocado Smoothie

Prep time: 5 minutes

Cooking time: 3 minutes

Servings: 4

Nutrients per serving:

Carbohydrates – 17 g

Fat – 39 g

Protein – 5 g

Calories – 409

Ingredients:

- ½ cup full-fat coconut milk
- ½ cup coconut water
- ½ avocado
- ¼ cup baby spinach
- 1 handful fresh parsley
- 1 drop stevia extract

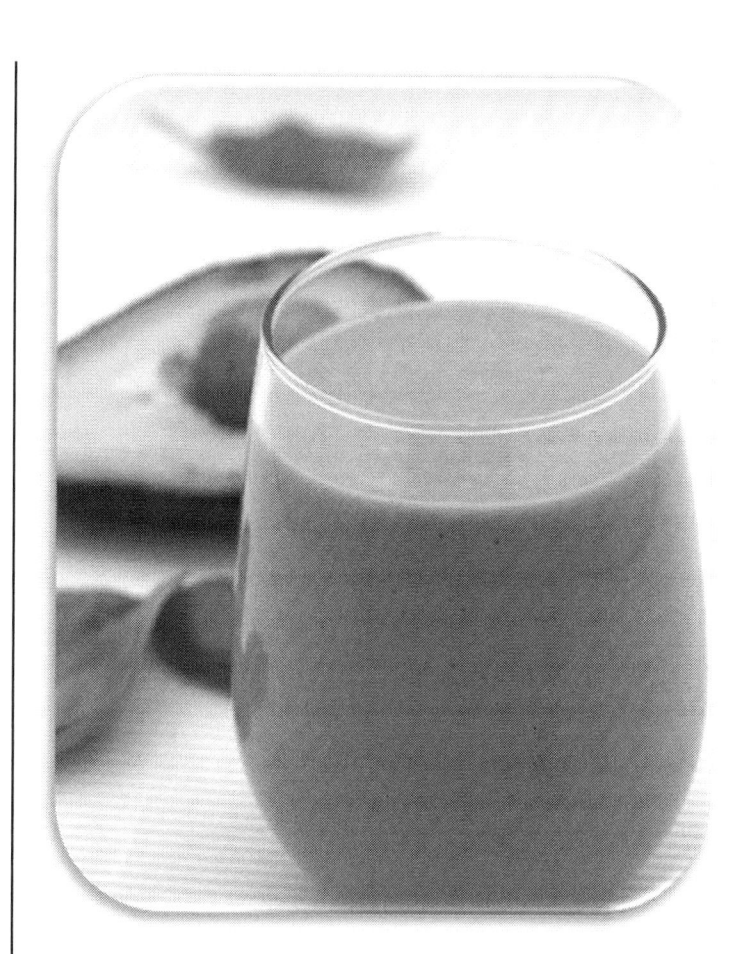

Instructions:

1. Combine all the ingredients in a blender and mix until smooth.
2. Enjoy your tasty smoothie!

High Protein Blueberry Banana Smoothie

Prep time: 5 minutes

Cooking time: 5 minutes

Servings: 2

Nutrients per serving:

Carbohydrates – 17 g

Fat – 39 g

Protein – 5 g

Calories – 388

Ingredients:

- 1 cup blueberries, frozen
- 2 ripe bananas
- 1 cup water
- 1 tsp vanilla extract
- 2 Tbsp chia seeds
- ½ cup cottage cheese
- 1 tsp lemon zest

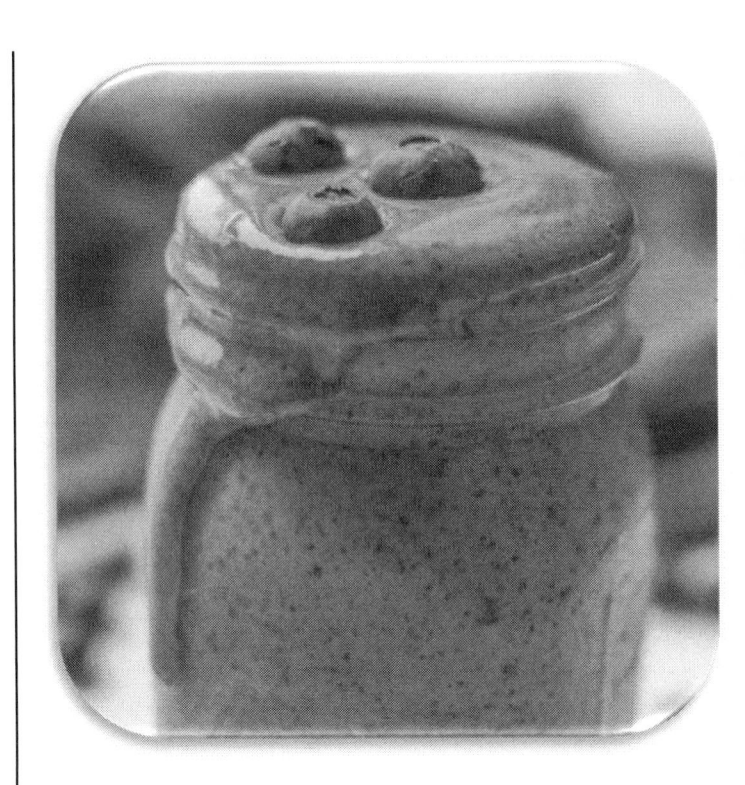

Instructions:

1. Put all the smoothie ingredients into the blender and whisk until smooth.
2. Enjoy your wonderful smoothie!

Ginger Smoothie with Citrus and Mint

Prep time: 5 minutes

Cooking time: 3 minutes

Servings: 3

Nutrients per serving:

Carbohydrates – 39 g

Fat – 5 g

Protein – 6 g

Calories –206

Ingredients:

- 1 head Romaine lettuce, chopped into 4 chunks
- 2 Tbsp hemp seeds
- 5 mandarin oranges, peeled
- 1 banana, frozen
- 1 carrot
- 2-3 mint leaves
- ½ piece ginger root, peeled
- 1 cup water
- ¼ lemon, peeled
- ½ cup ice

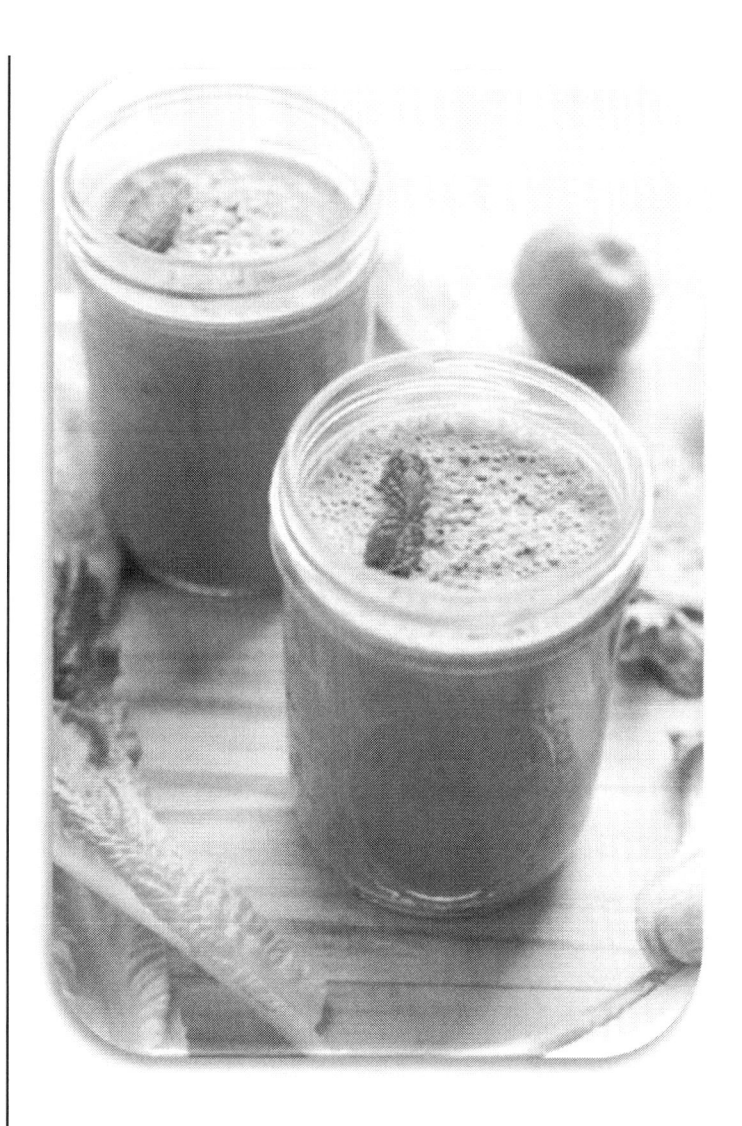

Instructions:

1. Put all the smoothie ingredients in a blender and blend until smooth.
2. Enjoy!

Strawberry Beet Smoothie

Prep time: 5 minutes

Cooking time: 50 minutes

Servings: 2

Nutrients per serving:

Carbohydrates – 44.4 g

Fat – 1.2 g

Protein – 4.5 g

Calories –191

Ingredients:

- 1 red beet, trimmed, peeled and chopped into cubes
- 1 cup strawberries, quartered
- 1 ripe banana
- ½ cup strawberry yoghurt
- 1 Tbsp honey
- 1 Tbsp water
- Milk, to taste

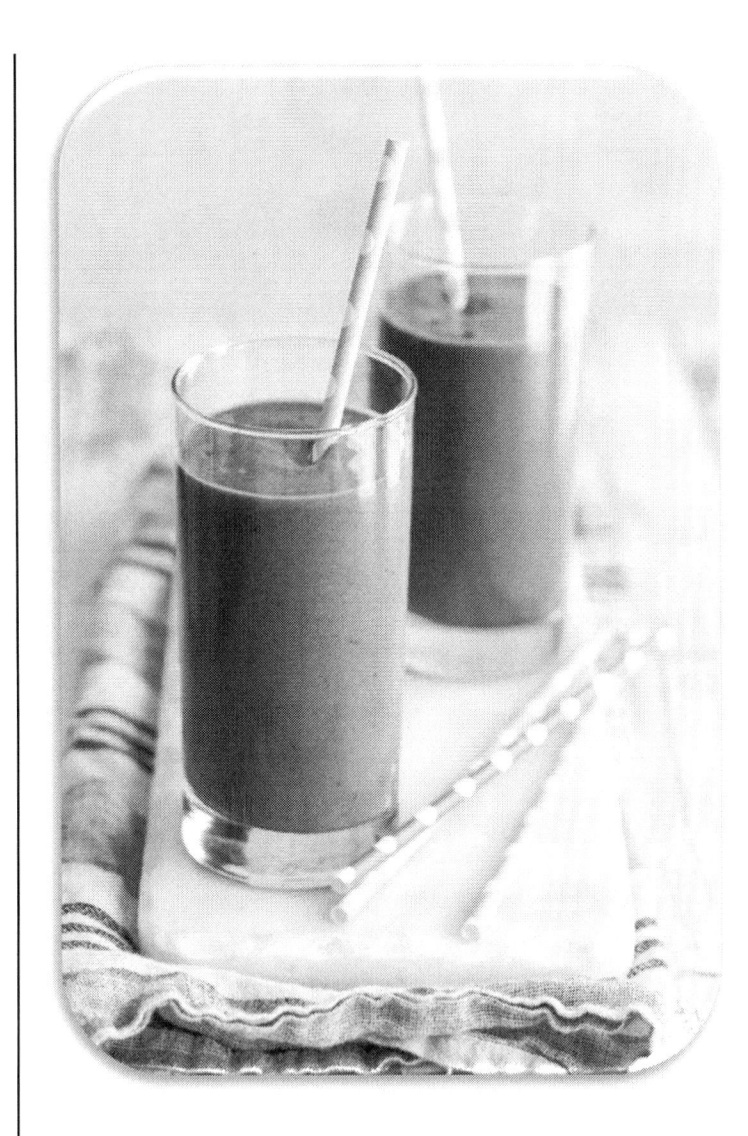

Instructions:

1. Sprinkle the beet cubes with water, place on aluminum foil and put in the oven (preheated to 204°C). Bake for 40 minutes.
2. Let the baked beet cool.
3. Combine all the smoothie ingredients.
4. Enjoy your fantastic drink.

Peanut Butter Shake

Prep time: 5 minutes

Cooking time: 5 minutes

Servings: 2

Nutrients per serving:

Carbohydrates – 62 g

Fat – 11 g

Protein – 10 g

Calories – 361

Ingredients:

- 1 cup plant-based milk
- 1 handful kale
- 2 bananas, frozen
- 2 Tbsp peanut butter
- ½ tsp ground cinnamon
- ¼ tsp vanilla powder

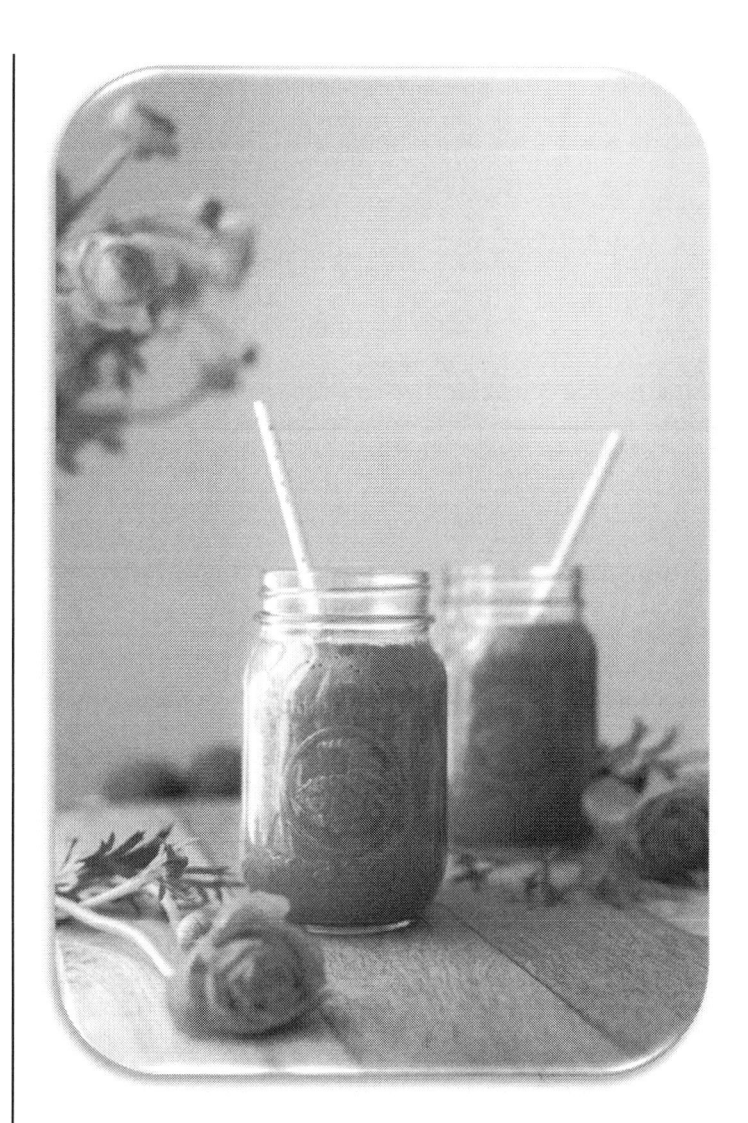

Instructions:

1. Use a blender to combine all the ingredients for your shake.
2. Enjoy it!

Chocolate Oatmeal Smoothie with Peanut Butter

Prep time: 5 minutes

Cooking time: 3 minutes

Servings: 2

Nutrients per serving:

Carbohydrates – 56.7 g

Fat – 16.7 g

Protein – 14 g

Calories – 427

Ingredients:

- ½ cup quick 1-minute oats
- 1 cup ice cubes
- 1 cup unsweetened coconut milk
- 2 Tbsp peanut butter
- 1 Tbsp cocoa powder
- 1 Tbsp honey
- 1 tsp vanilla extract

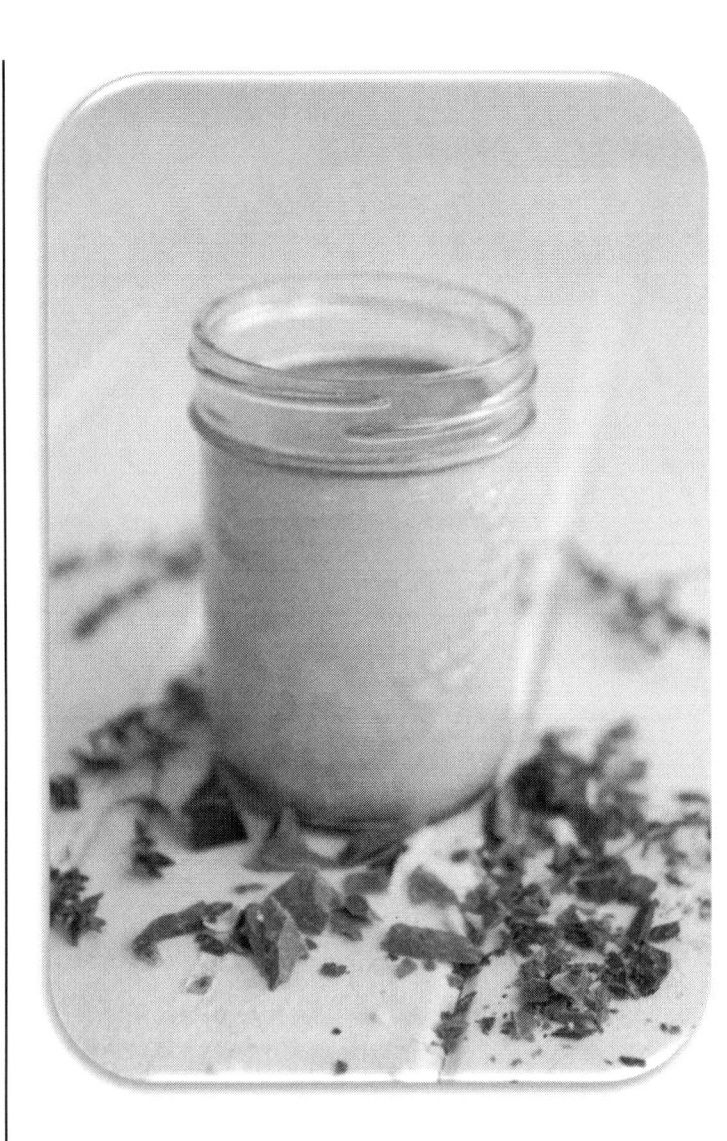

Instructions:

1. Use a blender to make the oatmeal powder.
2. Combine all the smoothie ingredients with the oatmeal powder and blend until smooth.

Hearty Peach Shake

Prep time: 5 minutes

Cooking time: 3 minutes

Servings: 2

Nutrients per serving:

Carbohydrates – 58 g

Fat – 5 g

Protein – 12 g

Calories – 313

Ingredients:

- ½ cup old-fashioned oats
- 2 cups peach slices, frozen
- 1 cup vanilla yoghurt
- ½ cup milk
- 1 Tbsp honey
- ¼ tsp vanilla extract
- ¼ tsp cinnamon
- Additional milk (if needed)

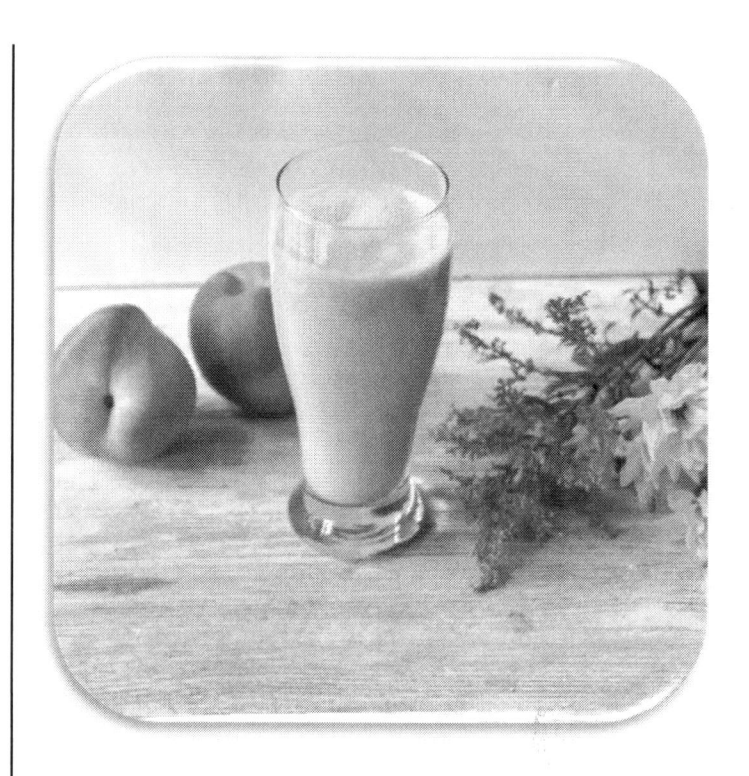

Instructions:

1. Blend the oats and add all the remaining ingredients to the blender. Blend until the mixture becomes smooth.
2. Serve and enjoy your smoothie!

CONCLUSION

Thank you for reading this book and having the patience to try the recipes.

I do hope that you have had as much enjoyment reading and experimenting with the meals as I have had writing the book.

If you would like to leave a comment, you can do so at the Order section->Digital orders, in your Amazon account.

Stay safe and healthy!

Recipe Index

A

Almond Oat No-Bake Energy Balls 39
Apple Dutch Pancake 63
Avocado Toasts with Hummus 23
Awesome Chocolate Mousse 70

B

Baked Banana with Almond Butter 65
Baked Eggs with Herbs 15
Bell Pepper Salsa 28
Bell Peppers and Hummus 34
Bracing Coffee Smoothie 71
Breakfast Egg Muffins 18
Broad Bean Salad with Barley and Mint 46
Broccoli Pesto Fusilli 58
Buddha Mix 25
Bulgar Wheat Salad with Chickpea and Pepper 45

C

California Sandwich with Grilled Veggies 40
Chocolate Oatmeal Smoothie with Peanut Butter 80
Chunky Chickpea Soup 51
Coconut Muffins 68
Coffee Breakfast Pudding 20
Cold Cucumber Soup with Dill 53
Corn Pasta with Brown Butter 30
Cream Cheese Leek Risotto 57
Crispy Cheese Sticks 33
Crunchy Roasted Edamame 37

D

Delicate Banana Pancakes 64

E

Egg-Free French Toasts 19

F

Fresh Tomato Avocado Soup with Basil 54

G

Ginger Smoothie with Citrus and Mint 77
Greek Cheese Sandwich 43
Green Chickpea Flour Pancakes 16
Grilled Cheese Sandwich 41

H

Hearty Peach Shake 81
Hearty Potato Stew 55
High Calorie Oatmeal with Cinnamon 22
High Protein Blueberry Banana Smoothie 76

I

Indian Stew with Peanut 56
Inspirational Orange Smoothie 74

L

Lemon Mint Dressing 50
Lentil Bowl with Tomatoes and Garlic 27
Lentil Salad with Avocado and Feta 47
Linguine with Mushrooms 60
Low-Calorie Kale Chips 36

M

Maroccan Carrot Soup with Cilantro 52

N

Noodles with Carrot and Seasame 59

O

Oatmeal with Almonds and Cherry 21

P

Peanut Butter Shake 79
Pearl Couscous with Lemon 29
Perfect Movie Popcorn 35
Potato Chips 32

R

Raspberry Vanilla Cream 67

S

Sandwich with Egg Salad 42
Simple Avocado Smoothie 75
Simple Garlic Bread Snack 31

Soft Tahini Dressing 49
Spicy Veggie Wrap 26
Splendid Cherry Ice-Cream 69
Strawberry Beet Smoothie 78
Strawberry Cheesecake Toasts 66
Strawberry Grapefruit Smoothie..............73
Student Tomato Omelet 17
Sushi with Peanut Butter and Jelly..........62

T

Toasted Pumpkin Seeds 38

Tri-Colored Lunch Bowl..........................24

V

Vitamin Green Smoothie 72

W

Warm Salad with Cauliflower 48
Wild Rice Salad with Pomegranate, Pistachio and Persimmon 44

Conversion Tables

VOLUME EQUIVALENTS (LIQUID)

US STANDARD	US STANDARD (OUNCES)	METRIC
2 tablespoons	1 fl. oz.	30 mL
¼ cup	2 fl. oz.	60 mL
½ cup	4 fl. oz.	120 mL
1 cup	8 fl. oz.	240 mL
1½ cups	12 fl. oz.	355 mL
2 cups or 1 pint	16 fl. oz.	475 mL
4 cups or 1 quart	32 fl. oz.	1 L
1 gallon	128 fl. oz.	4 L

OVEN TEMPERATURES

FAHRENHEIT (°F)	CELSIUS (°C) APPROXIMATE
250 °F	120 °C
300 °F	150 °C
325 °F	165 °C
350 °F	180 °C
375 °F	190 °C
400 °F	200 °C
425 °F	220 °C
450 °F	230 °C

VOLUME EQUIVALENTS (LIQUID)

US STANDARD	METRIC (APPROXIMATE)
⅛ teaspoon	0.5 mL
¼ teaspoon	1 mL
½ teaspoon	2 mL
⅔ teaspoon	4 mL
1 teaspoon	5 mL
1 tablespoon	15 mL
¼ cup	59 mL
⅓ cup	79 mL
½ cup	118 mL
⅔ cup	156 mL
¾ cup	177 mL
1 cup	235 mL
2 cups or 1 pint	475 mL
3 cups	700 mL
4 cups or 1 quart	1 L
½ gallon	2 L
1 gallon	4 L

WEIGHT EQUIVALENTS

US STANDARD	METRIC (APPROXIMATE)
½ ounce	15 g
1 ounce	30 g
2 ounces	60 g
4 ounces	115 g
8 ounces	225 g
12 ounces	340 g
16 ounces or 1 pound	455 g

Other Books by Tiffany Shelton

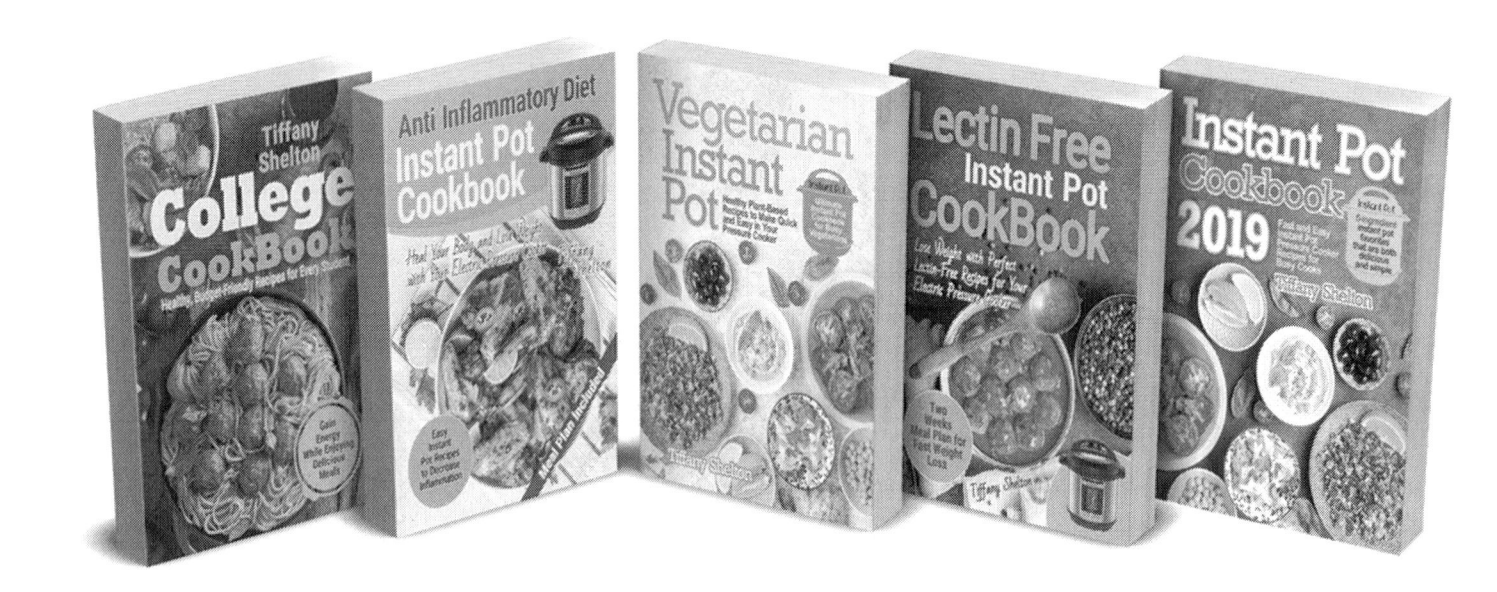

Tiffany Shelton's page on Amazon

Printed in Great Britain
by Amazon